4⁰⁰

D1053124

The
Healing
Power of
Touch

The Many Ways Physical Contact Can Cure

KARIN HORGAN SULLIVAN
CONSULTANT: ELLIOT GREENE

PUBLICATIONS INTERNATIONAL, LTD.

Karin Horgan Sullivan is a freelance journalist who specializes in health and alternative medicine. She writes the nationally syndicated newspaper column "Alternative Therapies," published by Universal Press Syndicate. Previously, she served as senior editor of *Vegetarian Times* magazine.

Elliot Greene, M.A., is former national president of the American Massage Therapy Association. He is "Nationally Certified in Therapeutic Massage and Bodywork" and has over 25 years experience as a massage therapist and workshop instructor. He was a major contributor for the National Institutes of Health's publication *Alternative Medicine: Expanding Medical Horizons*. Greene has been an expert advisor on massage therapy for numerous publications and serves on the Practitioners Advisory Panel of the *Journal of Alternative and Complimentary Medicine*.

Cover credit: **Bruce Ayres/Tony Stone Images**

Illustrations by Barbara Kiwak

Louis Weber, C.E.O.
Publications International, Ltd.
7373 North Cicero Avenue
Lincolnwood, Illinois 60646

Manufactured in China.

8 7 6 5 4 3 2 1

ISBN: 0-7853-2832-7

Library of Congress Catalog Card Number: 98-66644

Note: Neither the Editors of Consumer Guide™ and Publications International, Ltd., nor the authors, consultants, editors, or publisher take responsibility for any possible consequences from any treatment, procedure, exercise, dietary modification, action, or application of medication or preparation by any person reading or following the information in this book. The publication of this book does not constitute the practice of medicine, and this book does not attempt to replace your physician or your pharmacist. Before undertaking any course of treatment, the authors, consultants, editors, and publisher advise the reader to check with a physician or other health care provider.

CONTENTS

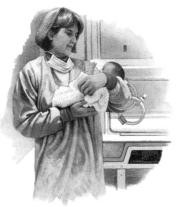

INTRODUCTION

In 1993, *The New England Journal of Medicine* published what proved to be a watershed article called "Unconventional Medicine in the United States." This study found that people were using alternative medical therapies in heretofore unimaginable numbers—just over a third of all adults in the country. Of the 16 interventions included in the study, touch therapy was among the most popular. Chiropractic ranked second only to relaxation techniques, and massage ranked third. Among the conditions for which touch therapy was commonly used were back problems, arthritis, sprains and strains, and headaches.

One of the study's most staggering findings was that people spent a total of nearly $14 billion on these unconventional therapies—most of it out of their own pockets. Despite the lack of acceptance by the medical establishment, people were drawn to the healing power of touch, even at a high financial cost.

Although the achievements of high-tech medicine have been enormous—just consider its life-saving ability to eradicate infectious disease—clearly it doesn't fulfill all of people's needs. Swallowing a pill or submitting to an invasive surgical procedure just doesn't feel as nurturing as the warm and caring touch of a massage. Not that the success of touch therapy is due simply to people's perception that it feels good; as you'll see in the next chapter, scientific research shows that it has a number of physiological benefits and is indeed a valid treatment for many ailments.

The aim of this book is to introduce you to the many varieties of touch therapy. Some of these therapies, mainly those that originated in Asia, date back several centuries and are steeped in tradition. A number of newer modalities developed in response to conventional medicine's failure to adequately remedy some ailments.

Though they differ in origin and particulars, these touch therapies have in common a fundamental belief in the body as a self-healing organism. Practitioners of alternative medicine, including touch therapists, take the approach that they aren't trying to cure a particular symptom. Instead, their goal is to help stimulate the body's natural inclination to heal itself, encouraging health on a more fundamental and lasting level than can be achieved by merely attacking and covering up symptoms, as many drugs do.

This book is divided into several sections. "The Power of Touch" explores the nature of touch and why it's essential to our well-being. The next section takes a detailed look at 30 different types of touch therapy, which have been divided into 10 categories. Here's a breakdown and brief overview of those categories.

Applied Kinesiology

Applied kinesiology is more of a diagnostic tool than a therapy.

The theory behind the practice is that the body knows why it is ill and reflects that knowledge in the muscles. By testing the strength of various muscles, a practitioner is able to diagnose imbalances in a person's health.

Biofield Therapeutics

A modality that defies easy categorization, biofield therapeutics—also called energy healing—blends ancient metaphysical tenents with modern-day physics. Energy medicine relates to many cultures' traditional belief that there is a universal life force that surrounds and flows through all of us; illness is a symptom of blockage or imbalance in the flow of this energetic force. Redirecting or altering the flow of energy enables the body to restore itself to health. Therapies included in this category are polarity therapy, reiki, and Therapeutic Touch.

Chiropractic

No doubt about it: Chiropractic is the king of touch therapies. In fact, chiropractic is the largest system of complementary medicine in the West and the third largest Western system overall, after standard medicine and dentistry. The premise behind chiropractic is that the natural state of the body is good health and that misalignment of the spinal column is a primary cause of pain and disease. By adjusting the vertebrae, the spine is realigned and the body is then able to bring itself back into balance.

Contemporary Western Massage

Contemporary Western massage encompasses a wide variety of techniques. This category includes a range of therapies, including aromatherapy massage, infant massage, manual lymph drainage, medical massage, myofascial release, on-site massage, sports massage, trigger point therapy, and reflexology.

Craniosacral Therapy

From the time a person passes through the birth canal, the head suffers a variety of traumas, from minor bumps and bruises to sharp blows. These injuries can disrupt the function of the craniosacral system, composed of the head and spine. Craniosacral therapy aims to correct abnormalities in this system, which improves both specific dysfunctions and overall health. The ability to find craniosacral imbalances is finely tuned; the pressure applied by the practitioner is rarely more than the weight of a nickel.

Oriental/Eastern Massage

Hands-on therapies go back thousands of years in countries throughout Asia, including China, Japan, and India. Therapies in this category include acupressure, Ayurvedic massage, Jin Shin Do, Jin Shin Jyutsu, shiatsu, and tui-na. Though individual practices vary in their specifics, they have in common a fundamental belief in a universal life force that flows through every living being. Stagnation or weakness in this energy leads to illness, while free-flowing, balanced energy creates good health.

Osteopathic Medicine

Osteopathic medicine can be a good place to start an exploration of complementary medicine, because it combines conventional and complementary approaches. Osteopathic physicians are qualified to provide the full range of medical services an M.D. is—such as prescribing drugs and performing surgery—but they're trained to take a holistic approach, one that favors using non-invasive, hands-on techniques. To stimulate the body's self-healing abilities, osteopathic physicians rely on physical manipulation to correct structural problems.

Physical Therapy

Physical therapy has always been a hands-on profession, dedicated to restoring physical function in patients with a wide variety of ailments, from birth defects to sports injuries. Physical therapists have a number of modalities at their disposal, including joint mobilization, electrical stimulation, and therapeutic massage.

Increasingly, though, physical therapy practitioners are going beyond the traditional techniques of their trade to incorporate more alternative touch therapies, such as acupressure, craniosacral therapy, and the Alexander Technique.

Structural and Functional Techniques

This category covers the Alexander Technique, Aston-Patterning, Feldenkrais Method, Hellerwork, Rolfing, and the Trager Approach. A combination of movement and physical touch, the therapies that fall under this umbrella— also known as movement re-education—teach patients how to use their bodies more efficiently. Unlike physical exercise and posture routines, which impose a mechanical reshaping of the body, movement re-education shows students that the ways in which they move can cause problems. Movement reduction then teaches them more beneficial movement patterns, which in turn relieve pain, stress, and fatigue.

Traditional European Massage

When most people think of massage, they think of the classic Swedish massage, which is perhaps the most popular form of bodywork in the world. A deeply relaxing therapy, Swedish massage is the foundation for many techniques of contemporary Western massage. And it does more than calm the mind: Research shows it alleviates pain, eases nausea, boosts immunity, and increases weight gain in premature infants.

Following "Therapies" is a section called "Conditions,"

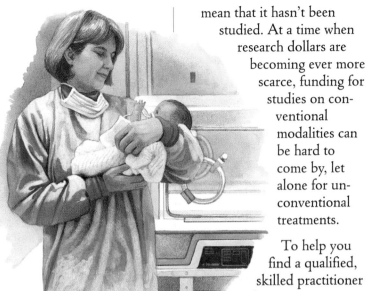

mean that it hasn't been studied. At a time when research dollars are becoming ever more scarce, funding for studies on conventional modalities can be hard to come by, let alone for unconventional treatments.

To help you find a qualified, skilled practitioner whom you can trust, we've provided the section "Choosing a Practitioner." It details the qualifications to look for and questions you should ask before establishing a relationship with a provider.

which covers more than 50 specific medical conditions that may be alleviated by touch therapy. For each of these we include a profile of the condition as well as the conventional approach to treatment. We also provide a listing of touch therapies that may be beneficial, as well as helpful self-care tips. Where scientific studies documenting a therapy's benefits are available, we've mentioned them, too. However, keep in mind that the efficacy of many of these therapies has not been scientifically proven. That doesn't necessarily mean that a particular therapy doesn't work though; it may simply

Taking advantage of touch's therapeutic benefits needn't always mean going to a practitioner. Giving a massage is one of the nicest things family and friends can do for one another. In "How to Give a Massage," we outline simple, straightforward guidelines for nurturing another person with touch.

Finally, a complete appendix provides a detailed listing of organizations to contact for more information.

THE POWER
OF TOUCH

T HE CHINESE
first wrote about massage over 4,000 years ago in
The Yellow Emperor's Classic of Internal
Medicine, the oldest Chinese medical text. (It
recorded practices of the emperor, who was believed
to have been born around 2700 B.C.) In the fourth
century B.C., Hippocrates, the Greek physician and
father of modern medicine, wrote that physicians
"must be experienced in many things, but most
assuredly rubbing." Throughout the millennia,
touch was the most important diagnostic and
therapeutic tool in the doctor's handbag.

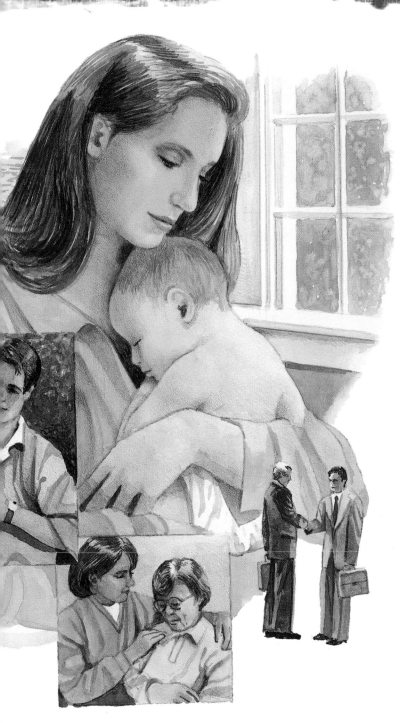

TOUCH

Touch therapy is one of the oldest forms of healing in the world, as old as humans' natural instinct to rub the spot that hurts. Anthropologists have found cave paintings in the Pyrenees mountains that depict healing with touch and have been dated all the way back to 15,000 B.C.

MODERN TOUCH THERAPY

Much of touch therapy as we know it in this country is rooted in Swedish massage, which was developed in the early 1800s by Swedish fencing master and gymnastics instructor Per Henrik Ling. Ling sought to create a type of body manipulation that echoed the benefits of Swedish gymnastics, an exercise regimen of 800 movements that increased circulation and muscle tone and balanced the body.

Like many other healers throughout history, Ling's interest in massage was due in part to having a health problem himself: The bodywork he created—which he called the Swedish Movement Cure—relieved his rheumatism. The Swedish government was less than enthusiastic about Ling's therapy, however. When in 1812 he applied for a license to teach his technique, the govern-ment rejected his request. Nevertheless, popular demand for Ling's treatment was so great that two years later his application was granted and began to be accepted by the Swedish medical and scientific establishment.

Therapeutic massage was introduced to the United States in the 1850s by physicians George and Charles Taylor. The brothers studied massage in Sweden, then returned home to New York and began using it in their practice.

In the 1870s, two Swedes were responsible for opening the first U.S. massage therapy clinics, one in Boston and one in Washington, D.C. The clinic near the Capitol attracted a number of famous clients, including Presidents Benjamin Harrison and Ulysses S. Grant. Swedish massage has remained the predominant type of massage therapy in the

The Healing Power of Touch

United States. Besides being the main therapy still taught in today's massage schools, its strokes can be found in aromatherapy massage, manual lymph drainage, and infant massage.

Hands-on techniques were once a standard part of doctor care, but that changed with all the wounded soldiers of World War I. Time-pressed physicians became less interested in hands-on healing and handed over massage duties to nurses and assistants. Also, the impact of drugs, anaesthesia, and other innovations gave medicine a greater emphasis on advanced technology. Eventually, most practitioners lost interest in massage. The therapy was left to a small number of therapists to continue the practice until the late 1960s and early 1970s, when natural medicine slowly began to experience a revival.

This rebirth was largely an outgrowth of the counterculture, which was characterized by questioning authority and openness to new ideas, as well as an ecological worldview that emphasized the importance of nature and humans' connection to it. Renewed interest in massage in particular was kindled by the human potential movement. At the heart of this movement was the belief that the most important source of authority was within the individual. Adherents were encouraged to deeply explore their feelings, not simply to get at the root of any dysfunctional behavior or neuroses but primarily for the purpose of self-development and achievement of one's highest potential. Encounter groups, primal-scream therapy, and "rebirthing" all came out of the human potential movement.

At the hub of the movement was the Esalen Institute in Big Sur, Calif., a personal growth center that offered (and still offers) a large program of massage instruction. Massage was emphasized as an important means of self-development. As taught at Esalen, both giving and receiving touch was viewed as a kind of meditation, a way of becoming grounded and finding one's true self.

Among the many bodywork practitioners invited to teach at Esalen was Ida Rolf, who had received a Ph.D. in biological chemistry from Columbia University's College of Physicians and Surgeons in 1920. During the course of her research and informal studies, Rolf discovered the importance of fascia, the flexible connective tissue that envelops all the muscles and organs in the body. Fascia is what gives the body shape, because it holds everything in place.

Over a person's life, fascia typically becomes distorted from such things as physical injury, poor posture, and even emotional trauma. Fascia adapts to life's insults by shortening and thickening, and pulling bones, muscles, and organs out of position. To release these ingrained patterns of tension and imbalance, Rolf, who herself suffered from scoliosis and spinal arthritis, developed a form of deep-tissue massage that she called Structural Integration, popularly known as Rolfing. The hall-mark of Rolfing is what is called the Rolf line. In a properly aligned body, a straight line drawn from a person's head to feet should intersect with the midpoint of the ears, shoulder joints, hip joints, knees, and ankles. In a typical patient, however, a line drawn through these midpoints is curvy, indicating misalignment.

Rolf developed a basic treatment series that consisted of ten progressive sessions, each focusing on a specific area of the body and building on the work of the previous sessions. Before the series began, the patient was photographed in his underwear to help evaluate distortions in the Rolf line. After completion of the series, the patient was photographed again so the practitioner could assess changes. The results were astounding. Besides exhibiting more symmetry in their bodies, patients appeared to have lost pounds and grown several inches taller. Their breathing improved dramatically, and many looked several years younger. Moreover, many patients experienced tremendous emotional release and growth during their sessions.

During the 1950s and '60s Rolf taught her technique primarily to osteopathic physicians and chiropractors but was unhappy because they perceived Rolfing merely as an adjunct therapy and not as a comprehensive program for integrating the whole person. Rolf at last found a home for her teachings at Esalen in the late 1960s, where her approach had a revolutionary effect. Up until that time, there hadn't been any kind of medical model for massage. Swedish massage was generally considered a luxury, usually offered at spas; it felt good and made the skin glow, but it wasn't necessarily a means of healing. Massage also was associated with "massage parlors," barely disguised covers for prostitution that sprang up on the seedier sides of towns.

Rolfing changed all that, by introducing a medical model to massage. Rolf's approach was based on science, and she had a structured method of treat-ment. What bodyworkers had for the first time was a systematic approach that documented clinical outcomes and was repeatable time and time again. Moreover, clients not only experienced profound physical benefits but deep emotional change as well. It was a comprehensive, systematic route to self-improvement in mind and body—the ideal therapy for the times. Today, Rolfing endures as the grandmother of any technique related to deep-tissue work: myofascial release, trigger point therapy, other structural techniques—in other words, nearly anything that isn't Swedish or Eastern in origin.

Another major influence on the practice of touch therapy in the United States has been the influx of ideas from Asia, where hands-on healing dates back thousands of years. The principles underlying acupressure, for instance, can be found in *The Yellow Emperor's Classic of Internal Medicine*, a comprehensive text of traditional Chinese medicine that records practices believed to be more than 4,000 years old. Shiatsu, or Japanese finger pressure massage, grew out of Chinese concepts. And Ayurveda—a Sanskrit term that means "knowledge of life"—is the ancient system of medicine that has been practiced in India for thousands of years.

The introduction of Eastern medical practices to the United States can be traced to President Richard Nixon's visit to China in 1972. During the trip, James Reston, a writer for *The New York Times* and member of the presidential press corps, fell ill with appendicitis and had to have emergency surgery. Acupuncture afforded him great relief from the resulting pain, and his experience became famous after he described it in an article. Nixon organized an educational exchange of Chinese and U.S. medical practitioners, and acupuncture achieved a high profile in this country. While they have remained lesser known, acupressure, shiatsu, and Ayurvedic massage have ridden the coattails of acupuncture and grown in popularity.

Today, massage therapy is experiencing an unprecedented boom. According to the American Massage Therapy Association, Americans visit massage therapists 75 million times a year, at a cost of over $3 billion. Several forces are driving the growth in massage therapy, but the main one is our quest for wellness. As the Baby Boomers grow older, they are increasingly seeking out ways to maintain their vitality. Massage has become an important way to reduce stress and stay healthy.

The mainstream medical establishment also is again beginning to embrace massage therapy. One study found that more than half of primary-care and family doctors surveyed said they would encourage their patients to use massage therapy as a treatment for various disorders. No longer viewed merely as a luxury reserved for wealthy spa goers, massage is even being covered by some

The Healing Power of Touch

health insurers. And a growing number of employers are recognizing the toll stress takes on its employees and are bringing massage therapists into the workplace for on-site massage; satisfied customers include Reebok, American Express, AT&T, and Merrill Lynch.

THE IMPORTANCE OF TOUCH

Touch is as essential to our health as the air we breathe and the food we eat. Of all the senses, touch is the only one we cannot live without. People born without sight or hearing learn to compensate for the absent sense. Those who lose their sense of smell or taste—through injury, for instance—may find life to be less pleasurable, but they too learn to endure. Without experiencing touch, however, a person may literally perish.

This became painfully clear in the early 1900s, following publication of the book *The Care and Feeding of Children*, written by Emmett Holt, M.D., a professor of pediatrics at Columbia University School of Medicine in New York City. Holt was considered the supreme authority on child-rearing, the Dr. Spock of his day, and his best-selling book had an enormous influence. His edicts turned the idea of tender, nurturing care for babies completely upside down.

Holt declared that too much attention and handling spoiled children and appealed to their animal instincts. Instead, he said, parents must banish cradles and rocking chairs and stop cuddling their children. Babies were not to be picked up when they cried, and they were to be fed on a rigorous schedule, not whenever they were hungry.

At the time Holt's book was published, medical care in the United States was undergoing a profound shift. Natural, hands-on treatments such as homeopathy and naturopathy were falling out of favor as what was called biomedicine began to dominate medical practice. Caught up in a fervor for all things modern, upper-class, well-educated Americans in particular subscribed to the new philosophy of biomedicine, characterized by a reliance on surgery, drugs, and other high-tech interventions. Holt's methods were simply one more modern innovation to embrace.

Within a few years, however, doctors began noticing a strange increase in deaths among seemingly healthy babies, especially at "the best" orphanages and hospitals. In fact, at some institutions the mortality rate was nearly 100 percent. No cause of death could be determined; the children simply became withdrawn, lost weight, and died. Even more peculiar was that at a time when most childhood diseases were associated with poverty, which often went hand in hand with unsanitary living conditions, this phenomenon was associated with wealth. Stymied doctors called the disease marasmus, Greek for "wasting away."

Looking for answers, an American pediatrician named Fritz Talbot paid a visit to a children's hospital in Dusseldorf, Germany. Talbot was interested in the clinic because, although its pediatric medical practices were much like those in the United States, marasmus was virtually unknown there. As he toured the wards, Talbot's attention was caught by an elderly woman who was holding and caressing the children. The doctors explained that the woman was a nurse called Old Anna. When they had done everything they could for a baby, they turned it over to Old Anna for cuddling. Her treatment, they said, was always successful.

Suddenly, the mystery of marasmus was solved. Children were failing to thrive because they weren't being touched enough—at least in the upper classes. Holt's commandments hadn't trickled down to poor women, who continued to do as they'd always done and held, rocked, and comforted their children. As a result, marasmus was rare among the lower class.

Talbot went back to the United States and set off a backlash against Holt. He urged hospitals to encourage their staffs to "mother" pediatric patients, to pick them up and hold and rock them throughout the day. Once hospitals finally found the courage to reject Holt and listen to Talbot, the incidence of marasmus soon dropped dramatically.

EMOTIONAL BENEFITS

Touch isn't important to just physical well-being; research in the 1950s found that it's essential for psychological well-being too. Researchers conducted experiments with newborn Rhesus monkeys who were taken from their mothers and given access to two inanimate surrogate "mothers."

Both mothers provided milk for the baby monkeys to suckle. The difference was that one mother was constructed entirely of wire and the other was made of a soft padding. The monkeys showed an overwhelming preference for the padded mother, clinging to it, hugging it, and rubbing their bodies on it. When researchers frightened the baby monkeys, they ran to the padded mother, rather than the wire one, for comfort. And when the surrogate mothers were placed behind windows with sliding doors, the babies would even open the doors simply to stare at the padded mother.

The need for touch became even more apparent when the monkey babies were given access to only one surrogate mother. The monkeys with the wire mother became depressed, neurotic, and confused. Unlike the monkeys with the padded mother, who explored and played with abandonment, the wire-mother group sat huddled in the corner, morosely rocking back and forth.

A SENSE TAKEN FOR GRANTED

Despite the lessons we've learned about the importance of touch, today we are experiencing an intense skin hunger. As our world becomes increasingly high-tech, opportunities for in-person human contact continue to decline. Telecommuters spend their days working from home, where interaction with co-workers is kept to a minimum. We order clothing from merchants over the telephone, and a few days later it appears in the mail. Plane tickets can be purchased over the Internet without ever talking to a live human being. We make deposits and withdrawals of money at automatic teller machines. Dinner comes from a disembodied voice speaking through a "squawk box" at the drive-through line of a fast-food restaurant.

Though our everyday speech is riddled with references to touch—he's had a "touch of the flu," that's a "touchy sub-ject," she's a "soft touch"—most of us don't even notice the influence of this sense on practically everything we do. Think about the simple act of making yourself a piece of toast. As you take the package of bread off the shelf, your hand perfectly senses its weight and uses just the right amount of pressure to lift it, so that you don't toss it into the air. You feel the texture of the bread as you remove a slice—is it firm, bumpy whole-grain bread or soft, squishy white bread?—and you begin to salivate as you imagine what it's going to taste like. Your fingers sense the level of tension in the lever of the toaster as you push it down hard enough to make it stick but not so hard as to slam it. When the bread is toasted, you spread butter and jam on it; if the butter is cold—an-other touch sensation—you will need to hold the knife more firmly and use more pressure to spread it. When you take a bite of the toast, notice the way the bread has undergone a transformation and become warm and crunchy. You can feel the melted butter and the sticky jam on your tongue.

Unless we deliberately pay attention, we tend not to notice touch sensations. They have a

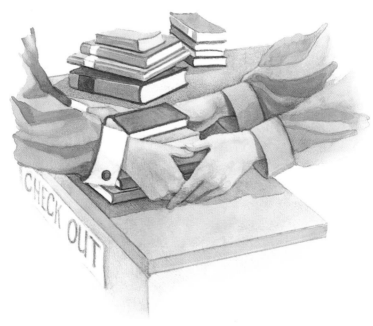

The Healing Power of Touch

dramatic affect on our unconscious mind, however, as a couple of interesting studies attest. In one study, researchers asked librarians to alternately touch and not touch people's hands as they returned their library cards to them. The unwitting subjects of the study were interviewed a few minutes later about their perceptions of the library—an object that doesn't normally elicit an emotional response. Those who had been touched reported feeling more positively about themselves, the librarians, and the library than the subjects who were not touched.

The results were rather amazing, given that the touch lasted less than a second and half the students didn't even remember being touched. In a similar study done in restaurants, waitresses who briefly touched patrons received bigger tips than those who did not.

HOW WE TOUCH

Why do we even have a sense of touch? At its most basic level, the sense of touch helps ensure our survival. Millions of sense receptors in the skin alert us to heat, cold, pressure, and pain, warning us of impending danger. The pursuit of pleasurable touch sensations is another means of perpetuating the species: The genitals are among the most sensitive areas of the body.

The receptors in the skin come in different varieties that are sensitive to only one kind of stimulus; cold receptors, for example, do not respond to heat stimuli. Sensitivity to a certain stimulus is determined by the number of those receptors in a particular part of the body. The fingertips are particularly well endowed with receptors for touch discrimination and can detect a change of less than .002 centimeters on a smooth surface. However, they have far fewer pain receptors and are thus fairly insensitive to painful stimuli.

Signals from touch receptors pass along sensory nerves directly to the spinal cord. From there they are transmitted to the relay station in the brain known as the thalamus. Finally, they go to the sensory cortex, the region in the outer part of the brain where sensation becomes part of our consciousness. Touch receptors provide only raw data; it is up to our brains to interpret that data by comparing it to the entire catalog of our experiences. Over time we learn to distinguish the sensation of a piece of burlap or a piece of silk, hot tea or cold lemonade, the prick of a pin or the cut of a knife.

In recent years, researchers have begun to understand that, besides providing us with information about the outside world, touch causes a series of chemical changes within the body, leading to a number of beneficial effects on human health. Much of this research has been conducted by the Touch Research Institutes, founded in 1992 by Tiffany Field, Ph.D., a professor of psychology, pediatrics, and psychiatry at the University of Miami School of Medicine.

TOUCH FOR HEALTH

Field became interested in the benefits of touch in the mid-1970s, when her daughter was born prematurely. She knew about the research showing that monkeys deprived of maternal touch suffered psychological and physical problems. She wondered what effect the lack of touch might have on preemies, who are kept in isolated incubators.

Field set up a study in which one group of premature infants received three 15-minute massages a day, while another group of preemies did not receive any massage. Even though both groups had the same calorie intake, the massaged babies gained 47 percent more weight than the other babies. It was discovered that massage stimulated the infants' brains to release more insulin, which helped the babies' bodies use their food more efficiently.

The Touch Research Institutes have conducted more than 60 studies that have shown positive results from massage therapy, many of them for pediatric concerns. One of the most significant benefits of massage is that it causes the body to release endorphins, natural opiate-like chemicals that alleviate pain and produce a feeling of well-being.

The conditions that the Touch Research Institute has studied include the following.

❋ Pediatric sleep problems: After a month, nearly 70 percent of children who received 15-minute massages before bed experienced cessation of sleeplessness or nighttime waking, compared to only 30 percent of children who were simply read Dr. Seuss stories before bedtime.

* Asthma: Studies in asthmatic adults and children have found that massage reduces levels of cortisol, a stress hormone that can exacerbate asthma. Reduction of cortisol levels leads to lower anxiety, reduced symptoms, and decreased recovery time during an asthmatic episode.

* Juvenile diabetes: Nearly a third of diabetic children fail to fully comply with their treatment regimen of insulin therapy, diet control, and exercise. Diabetic children who received 15-minute massages from their parents before bedtime for a month showed decreased levels of stress hormone, improved compliance with insulin and dietary treatment, and lowered levels of blood glucose.

* Job stress: Adults who received 15-minute chair massages twice a week in their offices were more alert and performed better on math problems immediately after being massaged than subjects who merely took a work break. At the end of the five week study, subjects reported that they experienced reduced job stress and were less depressed overall.

* Eating disorders: Compared to subjects who received only conventional care, hospitalized adolescent eating-disorder patients who received massage experienced lower levels of depression, decreased levels of stress hormones, increased levels of dopamine (a neurotransmitter that improves mood), and improved attitudes about their illness.

* Pediatric atopic dermatitis: This chronic, inflammatory skin condition is one of the most common ailments among children. A month of 20-minute daily massages improved all symptoms of the disorder, including redness, scaling, itching, and thickening and cracking of the skin. In contrast, a group of children who received only standard dermatological treatment—mainly topical emollients and corticosteroids—experienced improvement only in scaling.

* HIV infection: Massage therapy increases immune function in patients infected

with HIV, the virus that causes AIDS. Subjects received 45-minute massages five days a week for a month. Compared to the control period, when they did not receive massage, patients experienced a rise in the number of natural killer cells (a vital indicator of immune function). Patients also had lower levels of cortisol, a stress hormone, and they reported feeling less anxiety.

* Fibromyalgia: Fibromyalgia is a rather mysterious disorder characterized by chronic, generalized muscle pain and stiffness that has no apparent cause. Sufferers who received 30-minute massages twice a week for five weeks reported reduced pain and stiffness, less fatigue, decreased depression, and less difficulty sleeping.

A variety of other touch therapies have been found to have benefits as well. Research has found that:

* Chiropractic spinal manipulation alleviates low-back pain.
* Reflexology reduces symptoms of premenstrual syndrome.
* Therapeutic Touch accelerates wound-healing.
* Acupressure reduces nausea from both pregnancy and cancer chemotherapy treatment.
* Rolfing relieves anxiety.

GETTING IN TOUCH WITH TOUCH

While various research findings have elevated the sense of touch to new heights, from survivalist protection to medical therapy, most of us would do well to enjoy touch at a level in between these two extremes, as a way to enhance our everyday lives. This likely won't be easy, given that studies have found Americans to be clearly touch-phobic. Research conducted by observing couples in cafes around the world found that people in Puerto Rico touched an average of 180 times per hour and in France 110 times per hour. In comparison, the rate of casual touch among couples in the United States was shockingly low—just twice an hour.

Tiffany Field of the Touch Research Institutes found similar results when she observed teenagers at McDonald's restaurants in Paris and Miami. French teenagers were very comfortable with casual touch, as they leaned on one another, touched each other's arms, and put an arm around their friends' shoulders.

In contrast, American teenagers avoided touching each other, instead engaging in rather nervous self-touch, such as twirling their finger rings and cracking their knuckles.

Clearly, these behaviors are part of children's cultural inheritance; French parents and teachers are far more physically affectionate, while in the United States, parents and teachers are much more reserved. The difference has profound social implications: Cultures in which children are touched on a more regular basis have lower rates of adult violence.

Perhaps these findings can be an impetus to become a more "touchy" society. Hugging a child, briefly touching the arm of a kind stranger, giving your mate a neck rub—all these types of touch can go a long way toward bringing us more peace and contentment in our daily lives.

TOUCH
THERAPIES

HEALTH CARE IN America is changing rapidly. Health care providers increasingly view patients as consumers of their services, and each person is being called on to accept the responsibility of making informed decisions about his or her own health. Each day brings reports of sophisticated new diagnostic techniques and methods of treatments, but this outpouring of information can be more overwhelming than it is reassuring. To take full advantage of this new era in medicine, you owe it to yourself and your family to learn all you can about the various touch therapies and the conditions they are useful in treating.

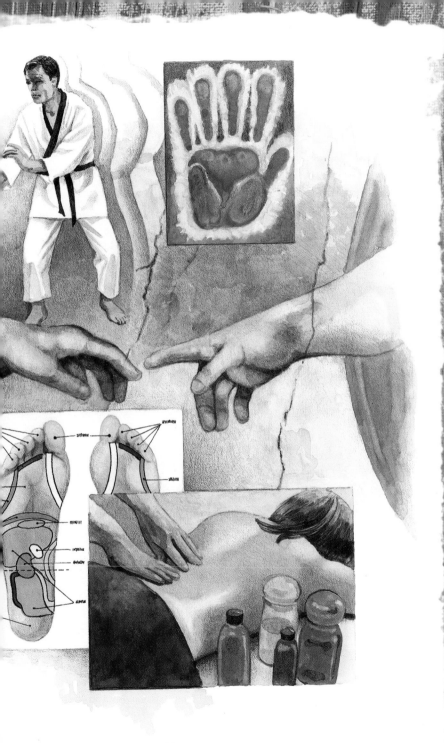

ACUPRESSURE

Acupressure is based on the same principles as acupuncture, but rather than inserting needles into certain points in the body, the practitioner applies finger pressure to the points. Because the majority of points are accessible to the patient, acupressure is an easily learned self-help technique for a variety of conditions, especially pain and nausea.

HISTORY

Given that our instinctive response to pain is to rub the spot that hurts, it's likely that a basic form of acupressure has been around since the beginning of humankind. The principles underlying acupressure came out of China and can be found in *The Yellow Emperor's Classic of Internal Medicine*, a comprehensive text of traditional Chinese medicine that records practices believed to date back more than 4,000 years. Acupressure actually predates the more well-known acupuncture, which is considered a higher-tech therapy because it uses needles.

The Western world received a formal introduction to tradi-tional Chinese medicine in the early 1970s, when President Nixon visited China. James Reston, a writer for *The New York Times* and member of the press corps on the trip, fell ill with appendicitis and had to have emergency surgery. Acupuncture afforded him great relief from the resulting pain, and his experience became famous after he described it in an article. President Nixon organized an educational exchange of Chinese and U.S. medical practitioners, and acupuncture achieved a high profile in this country. While it has remained lesser known, the use of acupressure has accompanied the growth of acupuncture.

WHAT IT IS

Acupressure is based on the Chinese concept of *qi*, or *chi*, the vital life force that animates all living beings. *Qi* flows throughout the body along 12 main channels, called meridians, each associated with a particular organ. Disease is believed to be the result of either excessive or weak *qi*.

Practitioners can help balance the flow of *qi* by stimulating specific points among the hundreds of acupressure points located along the meridians and smaller channels called collaterals. The practitioner generally uses her thumbs, fingers, or knuckles to apply pressure to the points, and the pressure may be light or deep, depending on the desired affect. Applying pressure for less than ten seconds has a stimulating affect, whereas a longer time period—up to three minutes—is sedating.

Besides using finger pressure, a practitioner may also use tiny seeds to apply pressure to certain points. The seeds are taped into place, often on the ear, then pressure is applied. After a treatment session, the patient can continue to periodically stimulate these points himself by pressing on the seeds.

PUTTING THE PRESSURE ON

Acupressure is a simple technique that lends itself well to home-care for minor ailments. Here are some common problems and the points that may alleviate them.

* *Colds with congestion:* GB20, on either side of the spine at the base of the skull.
* *Headaches:* GB20, on either side of the spine at the base of the skull. LI4, on the back of the hands in the webbing between the thumb and index finger.
* *Menstrual cramps:* SP6, located four finger lengths above the inner ankles.
* *Nausea:* LI4, on the back of the hands in the webbing between the thumb and index finger. P6, on the inner wrists three finger lengths above the wrist crease. ST41, in the webbing between the second and third toes.
* *Temporomandibular disorder (TMD pain):* GB20, on both sides of the spine at the base of the skull; press both sides at once.

No one is certain why acupressure works, and scientists have not yet found a way to document the existence of *qi*. Nevertheless, researchers have used electrical devices to discover that acupressure points are points of high conductivity, that is, points where the skin is least resistant to electrical input.

Several theories offer possible explanations for acupressure's effects. One says that muscle tension that accumulates around acupressure points impedes circulation of both blood and *qi*. Acupressure helps alleviate the tension, causing an increase in circulation and release of toxins, which helps boost disease resistance. Another possible explanation is that acupressure causes the release of endorphins, a type of hormone that alleviates pain and produces a sense of well-being.

USES

Research has shown acupressure to benefit several specific conditions. Stimulating what is called the P6 point, located on the inner wrists three finger lengths above the wrist crease, alleviated nausea and vomiting in both chemotherapy patients and pregnant women. Applying ice to LI4, the point on the back of the hands in the webbing between thumb and index finger, cut dental pain in half in patients with abscesses and other dental problems.

Although acupressure can be very helpful in alleviating some of the discomforts of pregnancy, especially morning sickness, pregnant women should not use acupressure without the advice of a health care practitioner. Pressure on certain points can cause uterine contractions and lead to miscarriage.

Acupressure should also be avoided if you have a heart condition, after a heavy meal or exertion, in cases of acute infection, or on points where there is a bruise, open wound, mole, wart, or varicose vein.

WHO PERFORMS IT

A variety of hands-on practitioners may use acupressure, including acupuncturists and massage therapists. Acupressure is taught in some massage therapy programs. Many Asian cultures have their own forms of acupressure or pressure-point technique.

ALEXANDER TECHNIQUE

This system of bodywork puts particular emphasis on reshaping the relationship among the head, neck, and shoulders. With a large following in the field of performing arts, the Alexander Technique has become one of the most widely respected forms of movement re-education in the world.

HISTORY

Frederick Matthias Alexander, born in 1869, was a Shakespearean actor in Australia. He was quite successful but developed vocal problems that threatened to ruin his career. After losing his voice altogether, he consulted with many physicians and tried a variety of medications, all to no avail. Finally, though only in his early 20s, he was forced to retire from acting.

Alexander spent the next decade on a mission to understand the cause of his vocal dysfunction. Using mirrors, he studied his body as he spoke and recited, eventually noticing that there was a pattern of tension among his head, neck, and torso. He found that his habit of pulling his head back and down compressed his larynx. After many months of physically retraining his body to adopt beneficial patterns of movement, his voice came back.

This experience became the basis of the Alexander Technique, which he taught abroad, mainly in England and the United States. Unfortunately, many of Alexander's students died in World War II, and his work wasn't widely known until 1974, when Nikolaas Tinbergen, a biologist at Oxford University, won the Nobel Prize for Physiology or Medicine. Tinbergen, a student of the Alexander Technique, titled his acceptance speech "Ethology & Stress Diseases: An Examination of the Alexander Technique," and the success of the therapy rapidly became known around the world.

WHAT IT IS

Most of us are completely unaware of how inefficient and

improper many of our movements are. These unconscious patterns typically establish themselves in early childhood and become conditioned responses that are difficult to correct.

Alexander believed that the most important physical relationship is among the head, neck, and torso; how these three relate to one another influences the rest of our physical body. An elongated spine and neck with the head properly balanced on top allow freedom of movement throughout the body and can alleviate tight muscles and a variety of chronic pains.

Rather than focusing on an individual symptom, such as back pain or restricted breathing, an Alexander teacher looks at the whole patient, analyzing how he sits, stands, and walks. The teacher uses hands-on and oral instructions to guide the student into better patterns of movement. Some instruction is performed with the student lying on a padded table as the teacher uses her hands to guide awareness to areas of tension.

The Alexander Technique is based on three fundamental steps. First, students become aware of their patterns of movement and how they interfere with proper posture, balance, and coordination. After developing this awareness, students work to inhibit habitual patterns of movement before they happen. Finally, the focus is on establishing improved physical habits.

Because each person's way of moving is unique, the Alexander Technique is usually taught on an individual basis. A minimum of 10 sessions is recommended, and often as many as 30 sessions are needed.

USES

The Alexander Technique is not meant to diagnose illness or eliminate particular symptoms. Instead, teachers focus on retraining students to move properly, which, as a result, can have beneficial effects on various ailments. Benefits of the technique have been documented in a number of studies. It has been found to:

* Relieve chronic back pain
* Improve breathing

TEACHER TO THE STARS

The Alexander Technique is especially popular with musicians and actors, whose bodies must be in peak shape to perform well. Alexander himself trained many leading actors and actresses of the day, including the famous Lillie Langtry. Today, the Alexander Technique is part of the curriculum at many performing-arts schools, including the drama department at New York University, the Juilliard School, and London's Royal College of Music. Among the famous students of the technique are William Hurt, Kevin Kline, Paul Newman, and John Cleese.

* Lengthen neck muscles
* Improve posture
* Lessen anxiety and improve performance in musicians

Teachers of the Alexander Technique report that it also has helped:

* Neck and shoulder tension
* Arthritis
* Temporomandibular disorder (TMD)
* Headaches
* Gastrointestinal disorders

The process of gaining control over one's physical body and relieving physical tensions can have emotional benefits as well. Students report that the technique makes them feel calmer and gives them self-confidence and more energy. Elderly people often experience better balance and coordination. Athletes have used the technique to improve their performance.

WHO PERFORMS IT

The North American Society of Teachers of the Alexander Technique (NASTAT) is the main training and certification organization. NASTAT requires more than a thousand hours of training over a period of several years; the majority of training is hands-on practice. There are more than 1,500 Alexander Technique teachers around the world.

Applied Kinesiology

Applied kinesiology is more of a diagnostic tool than a therapy in and of itself. The theory behind the practice asserts that the body knows the reason it is ill and it reflects that information in the muscles. By testing the strength of various muscles, a practitioner is able to diagnose imbalances in a person's health.

HISTORY

George Goodheart, an American chiropractor, founded applied kinesiology in the 1960s. He began developing his theory while treating a man with a shoulder dislocation caused by a weak muscle. Goodheart applied deep pressure at the point where the muscle connected to the rib cage, and the problem disappeared.

As Goodheart worked on other patients, he found that massaging certain muscles strengthened seemingly unrelated muscles. Over time he developed a theory of energy circuits that connected various parts of the body—a concept similar to the traditional Chinese view that vital life energy, called *qi* or *chi*, flows along energy meridians throughout the body.

Besides being a chiropractor, Goodheart was skilled in a variety of other healing arts. He developed an eclectic treatment approach that incorporated acupressure, chiropractic adjustment, myofascial therapies, nutrition counseling, and herbal remedies. Goodheart's contributions were acknowledged in 1980 when he was asked to serve on the U.S. Sports Medicine Committee of the U.S. Olympic Team for the winter games in Lake Placid, N.Y.

WHAT IT IS

Applied kinesiology views the body as an integrated whole. A person's state of health involves a triangle of equally important factors:

* The structural side encompasses muscles, bones, joints, nerves, and organs.
* The chemical side includes nutrition and the effects of medicines and environmental toxins on the body.

* The mental side covers emotions, moods, and personal attitudes.

All these areas are interrelated, according to the theory; a dysfunction in one affects the two others. Applied kinesiology seeks to correct the primary imbalance, which then leads to improvement in overall health.

Being primarily a diagnostic art, the core of applied kinesiology practice is its examination techniques. To assess dysfunction, the practitioner applies pressure to what is called an indicator muscle, such as the thigh or biceps, while instructing the patient to try to maintain a certain position of a limb. If the patient is able to resist the pressure, the muscle is considered "strong"; if she can't, the muscle is "weak."

These muscle tests, called challenges, fall into three types:

* Physical challenge: If the practitioner suspects a structural problem, he applies pressure to bones as well as muscles.
* Chemical challenge: The practitioner tests for allergies and toxic reactions by placing foods and various other substances on the tongue or skin while testing various muscles.
* Mental challenge: The patient focuses on certain thoughts as the practitioner conducts muscle testing.

Goodheart created a chart showing that every muscle has an organ or gland associated with it. The theory is that a weak muscle indicates dysfunction in the organ that corresponds to that muscle. For example, lung problems show

TOUCH FOR HEALTH

An offshoot of applied kinesiology, Touch for Health was created in the 1970s by John Thie, a chiropractor and the founder of the International College of Applied Kinesiology. Although the college's official position is that applied kinesiology should be performed only by trained practitioners, Thie believed that it should also be taught to individuals as a self-help technique. The Touch for Health Foundation conducts workshops for laypeople, instructing them in how to conduct muscle and allergy tests and perform various physical exercises to balance overall health.

up as weakness in the deltoid muscle (the large muscle that covers the shoulder joint), whereas kidney disease manifests itself as a weak psoas muscle, near the base of the spine.

Applied kinesiologists also use standard diagnostic tools, such as clinical history, physical examination, and lab tests, as well as a specialized consideration of a patient's posture, gait, and lifestyle factors. Treatment tends to include a variety of hands-on therapies, such as acupressure, chiropractic adjustment, craniosacral therapy, and joint mobilization, as well as nutritional counseling and occasional herbal remedies.

USES

When he originally developed applied kinesiology, Goodheart used it primarily to diagnose and correct postural defects. Today, however, the practice has a more far-reaching goal: to maintain overall good health.

There have been few controlled studies of applied kinesiology, but practitioners say it can ward off a variety of degenerative diseases, including arthritis, cancer, diabetes, and heart disease. Presumably, these benefits are achieved by restoring good posture and range of motion, improving nerve function, and balancing the endocrine, immune, and digestive systems.

WHO PERFORMS IT

According to the International College of Applied Kinesiology, some laypeople and even practitioners perform muscle testing without adequate knowledge, which can lead to inaccurate diagnosis and inappropriate treatment. For that reason, the college recommends that patients seek applied kinesiology only from practitioners who are licensed to diagnose medical conditions—medical doctors (M.D.s), osteopathic physicians (D.O.s), and in some states, chiropractors and naturopathic physicians—and have been certified in applied kinesiology through their college.

AROMATHERAPY MASSAGE

Aromatherapy massage appeals to two of the most basic human senses: touch and smell. Scented oils enhance massage not only because they smell pleasant; research shows that they also evoke powerful emotional and physical responses, such as reducing anxiety and alleviating pain.

HISTORY

The art of aromatherapy—the therapeutic use of pure essential oils extracted from plants—is thousands of years old. Dating back to at least 4000 B.C., the ancient Egyptians used essential oils to embalm the dead. (The bodies of many mummies were fairly well intact when discovered by modern-day archeologists.) Cleopatra was famous for her plant-based perfumes, and Hippocrates, the ancient Greek known as the father of modern medicine, used aromatic plants to purge the plague from Athens.

Eventually brought to Europe by the Crusaders, essential oils were a regular part of medical care through the 1800s. Interest waned, however, as natural medicine was supplanted by drug- and surgery-based approaches.

Aromatherapy was revived in the 1920s by a French chemist named Rene-Maurice Gatte-fosse, whose family owned an essential oil-extraction business. One day when he was experimenting in the lab, Gattefosse burned his hand quite badly. He stuck it in a vat of lavender oil before rushing off to the hospital. By the time he arrived, his skin had already begun to heal. Eventually, he recovered com-pletely, without a scar. Gatte-fosse resolved to dedicate his life to researching essential oils.

Medical interest in the healing power of aromatherapy didn't take off until the 1960s, when a French physician named Jean Valnet published a watershed book in this area. Valnet had been conducting his own research in this area since World War II, when he used essential oils to treat wounded soldiers. Aromatherapy has since become part of some French medical school programs. The use of aromatherapy in medicine is widely used in other European countries as well.

The use of aromatherapy in massage was pioneered by another French scientist, Marguerite Maury. Seeking a way to use essential oils externally, she found that they were readily absorbed by the skin. Today in this country, aromatherapy massage has become extremely popular mainly for its pampering, relaxing qualities and is commonly performed at spas, but its heritage of treating illness should not be overlooked.

Tips for Using Essential Oils

Although essential oils are entirely natural, that does not mean that they are without side effects. Essential oils are extremely concentrated; 500 pounds of rosemary, for instance, produce just one pound of rosemary essential oil. Because they are so potent, certain precautions should be observed when using aromatherapy.

※ Never take essential oils internally. Some are toxic and can cause severe reactions, even death.

※ Do not use essential oils without the advice of a qualified health-care practitioner if you have a serious health condition.

※ Avoid essential oils if you are pregnant because some can stimulate uterine contractions and cause miscarriage.

※ Before using an essential oil, do a patch test to be sure it won't cause an allergic reaction. Combine about 12 drops of essential oil with four tablespoons of carrier oil, such as almond, apricot kernel, or grape seed oil. Swab a small amount on your inner arm. If you are going to have a reaction, it will be immediate. If you do experience redness or irritation, wash off the essential oil with straight carrier oil, which will remove it more effectively than soap and water.

※ When using essential oils for massage, always dilute them in a carrier oil to avoid skin irritation. Use about 12 drops of essential oil in four tablespoons of carrier oil.

WHAT IT IS

The essential oils used in aromatherapy are extracted from various parts of plants, including leaves, flowers, fruits, and roots. The composition of the oils is extremely complex and may contain several thousand different constituents. The therapeutic effects of aromatherapy depend on the complicated interaction of these individual components; while synthetic oils are available (often labeled as "perfume oils" or "fragrance oils"), they are not as complex as pure extracts, and aromatherapy does not employ them.

The aroma of essential oils is critical to their healing effects. Fragrance molecules enter the nasal cavity, where they penetrate its olfactory membranes. Though the exact mechanism is not known, these molecules somehow stimulate the limbic system, which, in terms of evolution, is the oldest portion of the brain and governs our emotions, moods, and also our memories.

Using essential oils in massage enables the body to absorb them directly through blood capillaries that are close to the surface of the skin. For massage, essential oils are diluted in a carrier oil, for a couple of reasons: Essential oils are extremely potent and can cause irritation and allergic reactions if applied directly to the skin. Also, they tend to vaporize rapidly, and a carrier oil, such as almond or apricot kernel, helps stabilize them.

Aromatherapy can be used in any type of massage, but it tends to be incorporated mainly into Swedish massage or acupressure. The long strokes in Swedish massage help speed essential oils into circulation. Applying essential oils to acupressure points targets certain energy centers in the body.

USES

Though the clinical effects of essential oils are not well documented, their psychological effects have a great deal of research to back them up. And herbalists point out that centuries of empirical evidence support the therapeutic use of aromatherapy for a variety of conditions.

* *Acne*: One study found that tea-tree oil reduced lesions without causing dry skin.
* *Anxiety and stress:* Research shows that essential oil of lavender and neroli (also known as orange blossom)

are adept at inducing a state of calm. Chamomile, melissa, clary sage, and rose also are used to ease stress.

* *Bacterial infections:* Tea-tree and lavender oils have proven antibacterial properties.
* *Depression:* Various citrus scents—most notably neroli, tangerine, and grapefruit—have been shown to ease depression.
* *Drowsiness:* Research shows that peppermint, basil, and clove can dispel sleepiness.
* *Headache:* One study found that a combination of peppermint and eucalyptus oils helped ease tension headaches.
* *High blood pressure:* Melissa, lavender, ylang-ylang, marjoram, and ginger help normalize high blood pressure.
* *Indigestion:* Ginger, peppermint, and fennel dispel gas and cramping.
* *Menopausal symptoms:* Clary sage, sage, anise, coriander, and cypress have hormone-balancing effects and help ease a variety of symptoms.
* *Menstrual cramps:* Chamomile, lavender, and marjoram help reduce cramping.
* *Nausea:* Ginger eases nausea caused by digestive problems and motion sickness.

* *Premenstrual syndrome (PMS):* Lavender, geranium, and rose alleviate a variety of symptoms.
* *Smoking cessation:* In one study, black pepper reduced craving for cigarettes.
* *Viral infections:* Lavender, lemon, thyme, and pine increase certain immune functions and can help fight viruses.
* *Varicose veins:* Chamomile, myrtle, and cypress may ease pain and inflammation.
* *Yeast infections:* Laboratory experiments found that chamomile, lavender, bergamot, and tea-tree inhibited about two-thirds of the growth of the yeast *Candida albicans.*

WHO PERFORMS IT

There is no formal certification for aromatherapists. Many massage therapists have taken workshops or studied it informally and incorporate it into their practice. Aromatherapy massage has become particularly popular at spas throughout the country. Aromatherapy massage is also suitable for home use, though certain cautions should be observed in accordance with the potency of the oils (see "Tips for Using Essential Oils," page 38).

ASTON-PATTERNING

Originally trained as a Rolfer, Judith Aston eventually disagreed with Ida Rolf's philosophy that the body should be symmetrical. Aston developed an approach that takes into account the body's natural imbalance in form.

HISTORY

As a girl, Judith Aston had always been fascinated by how people moved and how different one person's movements were from another's. She grew up to earn a master's degree in dance and became a dance and theater-movement instructor.

Just as her career was blossoming in the late 1960s, Aston suffered severe back and neck injuries in two separate car crashes. Doctors told her she would never dance again and urged her to have spinal fusion surgery. Aston decided to investigate whether alternative therapies could offer less invasive relief.

Aston's quest led her to the Esalen Institute, where Ida Rolf gave her the structural integration series, better known as Rolfing. The therapy afforded immediate relief and eventually restored full body movement. Aston became a student of Rolf, who asked her to develop a program that would help clients maintain the improvements created by Rolfing.

In the basic Rolf series, the therapist performs deep tissue massage that focuses on removing tension from the physical structure of the body; Rolf wanted to expand upon this basic principle by also eliminating tension from the physical function of the body, helping clients to move efficiently as they went about their daily lives. Over a period of five years, Aston developed the program now known as Rolfing movement integration, an essential part of the complete Rolf program.

Eventually, though, Aston disagreed with Rolf's notion that bodies should be symmetrical and straight. Because the two sides of the body are in fact never exactly the same, Aston believed it was important to take into account this asymmetry when showing clients how to move more efficiently. This fundamental disagreement led Aston to strike out on her own and develop Aston-Patterning.

WHAT IT IS

We all have unconscious patterns of movement that are as unique to us as our signature. These habits typically establish themselves early in life, as a result of physical activity, injury, and even attitudes. A child who isn't allowed to express anger, for example, may develop a tight, cramped posture that he carries into adulthood. Typically, these habitual patterns of movement are very inefficient, causing us to lose our natural-born grace and creating tension and pain throughout the body.

As with other types of movement re-education, Aston-Patterning is generally taught in one-on-one sessions. The therapist takes a detailed case history, and clients are often videotaped as they go about their daily activities, to help them clearly see where tension is created by how they sit, stand, walk, and perform tasks.

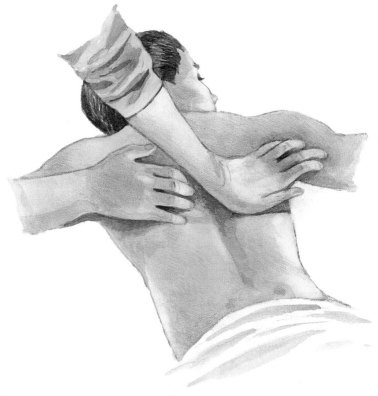

Besides showing patients how to move in ways that decrease physical tension, practitioners of Aston-Patterning also use massage to help release physical stress. Fundamental to Aston-Patterning bodywork is a spiraling technique that massages with the grain of the muscle, not against it. While one hand moves up the muscle, the other moves down in an asymmetric spiraling motion. This creates slack in the tissue that allows the practitioner to massage muscles deeply without causing the patient pain. Advanced Aston-Patterning applies a similar technique, called *arthrokinetics*, that allows deep massage of joints.

Sessions also include ergonomic training, which teaches clients how to restructure their home and work environments—for example, adjusting the height of a chair to reduce wrist strain while working on the computer. Finally, fitness training helps stretch and tone muscles and improve overall cardiovascular function.

USES

Controlled studies of Aston-Patterning have not been done, but practitioners say it can benefit just about anyone who wants to increase his physical poise. It's especially helpful for back and neck pain, posture problems, and other pain brought on by mechanical dysfunction, such as carpal tunnel syndrome. Those who do a lot of physical work, such as carpenters, dancers, and athletes, can also benefit from this form of movement re-education.

WHO PERFORMS IT

To become certified in the Aston-Patterning technique, a practitioner must complete a program taught at the Aston Training Center in Incline Village, Nevada. A listing of certified teachers is available from the center (see Appendix).

Ayurvedic Massage

Ayurveda is the ancient system of medicine that has been practiced in India for thousands of years. *Ayu* (life) and *veda* (knowledge) are Sanskrit terms that together mean "knowledge of life" or "science of longevity." Ayurveda has become popular in the United States only since the 1960s. The concept was introduced here by Maharishi Mahesh Yogi, the spiritual teacher who instructed the Beatles and who brought Transcendental Meditation (TM) to the West. The best-selling books of Deepak Chopra, a physician in California and a former student of the Maharishi, have led to an enormous growth of interest in Ayurveda in this country during the past few years.

HISTORY

The Ayurvedic practice of massage was first described in the Ramayana, one of the two great epic poems of ancient India. In the Ramayana, exhausted soldiers received massages from beautiful maidens, then refreshed themselves by swimming in the river. Hindu temple sculptures often depict Vishnu, the god of preservation, receiving a foot massage. Doctors have referred patients to massage practitioners since Ayurvedic medicine began.

Today, massage is a ritualized part of everyday life in India. In large cities, massage men set up mats in public places for anyone who wishes to hire their services. Daily self-massage with sesame oil to reduce skin dryness and alleviate anxiety is as important a part of Ayurveda's preventive approach as eating well and getting adequate rest.

In rural areas, families practice a tradition of weekly massage. Children receive massages every day from infancy through toddlerhood. Then they enjoy massages once or twice a week until school age, at which point they are old enough to exchange weekly massages with other family members.

Massage also is integral to certain rites of passage in India.

Just before their wedding, couples receive ceremonial massages with fragrant oils, to increase the bride's beauty and the groom's virility. A new mother also receives massage every day for 40 days after giving birth, to help purify her body.

WHAT IT IS

According to Ayurvedic principles, all of nature is governed by three fundamental life forces called *doshas*. From the moment of conception, each person has a constitution that remains unchanged throughout his life, known as the person's *prakriti*. This constitution comprises all three *doshas,* but one or two tend to predominate.

Following the lifestyle recommendations for your prakriti encourages good health. If, however, your lifestyle includes eating poorly, experiencing too much stress, or not getting enough sleep, one or more *doshas* becomes aggravated and illness occurs. The goal of Ayurvedic medicine is to bring harmony to the relationship among these *doshas.*

Season, time of day, climate, and diet are among other factors that can affect one's doshic make-up and throw it out of balance. Practitioners of Ayurvedic massage learn to assess patients' health by diagnosing their pulse, and they select different massage oils depending on which dosha is disturbed. Oil is essential to Ayurvedic massage and is believed to soften the skin, nourish the body, and improve overall health. Sesame oil is best for conditions caused by aggravated *vata dosha,* coconut oil for *pitta dosha*, and mustard or olive oil for *kapha dosha.*

Ayurvedic massage relies on four basic strokes that are similar to those found in Swedish massage:

* The practitioner begins by tapping the area to be massaged with cupped palms, to awaken the senses and increase circulation.
* Next, the area is kneaded, which removes tension, relaxing and softening the muscles.
* Rubbing the skin with oil lubricates the skin and evenly distributes body heat. It also stimulates circulation of lymph, the body fluid that carries white blood cells and is important to immunity.
* The fourth technique, squeezing, which is used only on the limbs, fingers, and toes, helps to increase circu-

lation to the extremities and release tension through the fingers and toes.

Practitioners also employ circular movements with their fingertips on pressure points called *marmas*. These points are located throughout the body and designate centers of the vital life force, known as *prana*. By deliberately holding a marma point with the thumb, the massage therapist can alter energy flow in the body.

USES

The primary focus of Ayurvedic medicine is prevention, and regularly receiving massage is considered a constitutional treatment that enhances and maintains good health. It relaxes the muscles and nerves, eliminates toxins, enhances breathing, induces deep sleep, aids digestion, and just generally makes life more pleasurable.

However, massage also can be therapeutic, and is often used to treat specific health conditions, including:

* General weakness, especially in invalids and the elderly
* Arthritis
* Rheumatism
* High or low blood pressure
* Sciatica
* Insomnia

During the first three months of pregnancy, Ayurveda holds that, along with certain yoga poses and breathing exercises, massage can strengthen the abdominal muscles and spine, which bear the weight of the developing baby. During the last six months of pregnancy, massage focuses solely on the back, to further strengthen the spine. At this time massage also incorporates relaxation exercises to help alleviate the intense emotional ups and downs that so often accompany pregnancy.

WHO PERFORMS IT

Though the interest in Ayurvedic medicine is growing in the United States, finding trained practitioners is still a challenge. Fully qualified Ayurvedic doctors typically complete a five-year medical program in India; massage therapists who use Ayurvedic practices may be found at Ayurvedic spas. Ayurvedic organizations may be able to provide referrals (see Appendix, page 244).

CHIROPRACTIC

Chiropractic is the largest system of complementary medicine in the West and the third largest Western system overall, after standard medicine and dentistry. The premise behind chiropractic medicine is relatively simple: The natural state of the body is good health and that misalignment of the spinal column is a primary cause of pain and disease. By adjusting the vertebrae, the spine is realigned and the body is then able to bring itself back into balance.

HISTORY

The origins of chiropractic can be traced back many centuries. Ancient healers from Asia, Greece, and Rome believed misalignment of the spine could be harmful to health, and Hippocrates, the father of modern medicine, advised healers to "get knowledge of the spine, for this is the requisite for many diseases."

Modern-day chiropractic was founded by Daniel David Palmer, a magnetic healer who spent nearly a decade studying anatomy and physiology before developing his theory that misaligned vertebrae could cause disease. He put his theory into practice in the 1890s when a janitor in his office building told him that he had become deaf 17 years earlier after throwing out his back. Palmer examined the man, found that one of his vertebrae was out of line, and adjusted it back into place. Within days, the janitor regained his hearing. Palmer went on to found the first chiropractic school, in Davenport, Iowa.

Chiropractors have fought a long, hard battle for acceptance from the medical establishment. Palmer himself was jailed for practicing medicine without a license, but his son carried on his teachings. In the 1960s, the American Medical Association (AMA) declared it unethical for physicians to associate with chiropractors and passed a resolution calling chiropractic an "unscientific cult."

Eventually, five chiropractors filed a restraint of trade complaint against the AMA. A federal judge ruled that the

AMA, along with the American College of Radiology and the American College of Surgeons, was guilty of conspiracy and of illegally boycotting chiropractors. The AMA fought the ruling, but it was upheld through years of appeals. Finally, in the late 1980s, the AMA lifted its ban.

WHAT IT IS

According to chiropractic theory, the body has an inborn inclination toward homeostasis and good health. The nervous system is critical to maintaining this state of balance: Nerve impulses travel from the brain to the spinal cord, then out to the rest of the body, helping it to grow and repair itself.

Problems occur when the vertebrae become misaligned, which can happen for a variety of reasons, including bad posture, injury, and stress. These misalignments—known in chiropractic as *subluxations*—interfere with the transmission of nerve impulses. If not corrected, over time this interference can cause pain and illness.

Chiropractors are trained to realign the vertebrae with rapid, thrusting movements called adjustments, or manipulations, which move vertebrae back

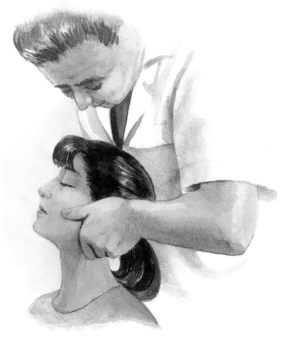

If you want to reduce your medical bills, you might want to give chiropractic medicine a try. A number of studies have found that for back pain, users of chiropractic care have lower health care costs than users of medical doctors, in part because they have lower in-patient treatment costs. Also, patients who miss work because of low-back pain are back on the job four times faster if they use chiropractic care than if they use standard medical care. And overall, chiropractic patients are three times more satisfied with their care than patients of family practice physicians.

into their proper positions. Chiropractic adjustments are not meant in and of themselves to cure illness. Rather, the emphasis is on supporting the body's natural tendency toward balance. Chiropractic adjustment allows nerve impulses to flow properly again, which, in turn, allows the body to heal itself.

The practice of chiropractic falls into two main categories: straight chiropractic and mixing. Straight chiropractic is narrow in scope, using only spinal adjustment to improve health. Mixers adopt a more holistic approach. Besides spinal adjustment, mixers employ a variety of adjunct therapies, including massage, applied kinesiology, acupressure, ultrasound, herbal medicine, nutritional counseling, and more. Neither approach is inherently better than the other; it simply depends on what an individual patient prefers.

USES

Because of its struggle for acceptance, the chiropractic profession for many years had difficulty getting its research published. In recent years, however, impressive results from chiropractic have been documented in studies published by the U.S. government and in the prestigious *British Medical Journal,* among other sources. Studies combined with anecdotal evidence suggest that spinal manipulation can help improve the function of the immune system, as well as ease arthritis pain, carpal tunnel syndrome, digestive problems, disk problems, jaw pain, menstrual pain, sports injuries, and whiplash. But two areas, in particular, deserve special attention:

Back Pain

Back pain is one of the most common ailments around; as many as 80 percent of Americans experience it at some point in their lives. You don't have to be elderly to suffer from it either; back pain is the leading cause of disability for Americans under 45. For years, the standard treatment for back pain was bed rest and painkillers, but a landmark study by the U.S. government found that spinal manipulation is the safest, most effective medical therapy.

A study of patients with debilitating back pain published by the *British Medical Journal* echoed this finding. In that study, some patients received treatment at a hospital outpatient facility, while others visited a chiropractor. Three years after treatment ended, the improvement in back pain was much greater in the patients who saw chiropractors.

Headaches

For years, anecdotal evidence suggested that chiropractic treatment relieved tension headaches, and a recent study backs this contention. The study compared chiropractic manipulation with treatment with an antidepressant commonly used for headaches. Though both groups felt relief during the treatment, the chiropractic group felt significantly better than the drug group a month after the study ended. Furthermore, most of the drug patients experienced unpleasant side effects from the medication, while virtually none of the chiropractic patients suffered ill effects from the manipulation.

WHO PERFORMS IT

Chiropractors obtain their doctor of chiropractic degrees—designated by the initials DC—from four- to five-year post-graduate programs in chiropractic medicine. Chiropractic physicians are licensed in all 50 states and the District of Columbia, and there are more than 40,000 licensed practitioners in the United States.

In order to become licensed, a chiropractor must pass written and oral exams. The scope of practice is fairly wide, though it varies from state to state. Some states, for example, allow chiropractors to order or even perform clinical lab tests, while others do not.

The Healing Power of Touch

CRANIOSACRAL THERAPY

From the time a child passes through the birth canal, the head suffers a variety of traumas, from minor bumps and bruises to sharp blows. These injuries can disrupt the function of the craniosacral system, composed of the head and spine. Craniosacral therapy aims to correct abnormalities in this system, which, in turn, improves both specific dysfunctions and overall health.

HISTORY

In the early 1900s, William Sutherland, an osteopathic medicine student in Kirksville, Missouri, had the idea that *sutures* in the skull—that is, the places where bones of the skull meet—are not fixed but flexible. For the next 20 years he studied this theory, observing that changes in suture position affected the brain and the pressure of the cerebrospinal fluid.

This fluid, which cushions and bathes the brain and spinal cord from skull to sacrum— the bone near the tail end of the spine that forms the back of the pelvis—is derived from the bloodstream and moves hydraulically. As the amount of fluid builds, pressure builds and moves the fluid up and down the spinal cord, at a rate of 6 to 12 cycles per minute.

Sutherland tested his observations with a variety of helmetlike devices that imposed sustained pressure on various parts of his skull. Different types of pressure produced different results. Some caused headaches, for instance, while others caused lack of coordination, and still others—according to his wife—caused personality changes.

Based on his studies, Sutherland created a system of examination and treatment that became known as *cranial osteopathy*. Because little was understood about how it worked and because the results at times seemed to be nothing short of miraculous, Sutherland's work was branded as cultist. Cranial osteopathy became an embarrassment to a profession that was struggling for mainstream acceptance, and in the mid-1970s, the Michigan State University Osteopathic College asked John Upledger, D.O., to either prove or debunk the therapy once and for all. Upledger's research team found that there was a solid scientific basis for Sutherland's work.

Upledger went on to develop craniosacral therapy, which is similar to cranial osteopathy. Whereas cranial osteopathy is oriented toward the bones, though, craniosacral therapy concentrates on the soft tissue, membranes, and fluid encasing the brain and spinal cord.

WHAT IT IS

Craniosacral therapists are trained to feel the wavelike motion of cerebrospinal fluid known as the *craniosacral rhythm*. Practitioners read this rhythm by placing their hands on the skull, the sacrum, and the coccyx, or tailbone, which all are attached to membranes encasing the fluid.

The ability to read the craniosacral rhythm is finely tuned; the pressure applied by the practitioner is rarely more than the weight of a nickel.

If the rhythm is weak—has a low amplitude—this a sign of low vitality and high susceptibility to disease. The practitioner also looks for symmetry in the rhythm, though lack of symmetry doesn't indicate exactly what the problem is but merely where it is located. A variety of abnormalities can cause disruption of the craniosacral rhythm, including dysfunction in the nervous, musculoskeletal, vascular, lymphatic, endocrine, and respiratory systems.

The therapist uses extremely gentle manipulation of the craniosacral system to correct imbalances. The goal is not for the practitioner to "fix" the problem, but rather to release tension in the system, which enables the body's inherent self-corrective tendencies to take over and restore itself to good health.

USES

There is not much published research on craniosacral therapy, but practitioners have used it to heal a wide variety of ailments:

VARIETIES OF CRANIOSACRAL WORK

There are three main types of craniosacral therapy:

✻ *The sutural method* is based on William Sutherland's original technique and focuses on manipulating skull bones at the places where they meet, called *sutures*.

✻ *The meningeal method* was created by John Upledger, the osteopathic physician who documented Sutherland's theories. This technique involves manipulating the membrane surrounding the brain, spinal cord, and cerebrospinal fluid.

✻ *The reflex method* is used by applied kinesiologists to stimulate nerve endings in the scalp, which relieves stress throughout the body.

There is also an advanced craniosacral technique called *unwinding*, which focuses on releasing specific trauma from the body by recreating the position of the body when the trauma occurred. Because physical trauma often causes psychological trauma, an unwinding session typically leads to emotional release as well.

✻ post-traumatic pain, particularly head and neck injuries
✻ temporomandibular disorder (TMD)
✻ headaches
✻ fatigue
✻ depression
✻ gastrointestinal complaints
✻ tinnitus
✻ sinus problems

Practitioners have also had success with pediatric patients, using it to treat dyslexia, hyperactivity, and cerebral palsy. Some craniosacral therapists even recommend using the technique on infants to help them recover from craniosacral trauma that occurs during birth from, for instance, the use of forceps or suction.

WHO PERFORMS IT

The Upledger Institute provides training in craniosacral therapy. A wide variety of health care practitioners use craniosacral therapy, including chiropractors, osteopathic physicians, physical therapists, and acupuncturists. In contrast, cranial osteopathy—the sutural method—is restricted primarily to osteopathic physicians.

FELDENKRAIS METHOD

Moshe Feldenkrais was well known for his work with patients suffering from neuromuscular disorders, such as cerebral palsy and multiple sclerosis. The Feldenkrais Method has helped patients gain motor control and increase mobility.

HISTORY

This form of movement re-education was developed by Israeli physicist and engineer Moshe Feldenkrais (rhymes with *rice*), who also is credited with introducing judo to the Western world. Feldenkrais was a martial arts student and an enthusiastic athlete who in the 1940s suffered a severe knee injury while playing soccer. Doctors told him that surgery offered only a 50 percent chance of recovery. Not liking those odds, Feldenkrais found a way to heal himself by applying his knowledge of anatomy, biomechanics, physics, and martial arts.

Despite the thousands of possible ways in which a person can move, Feldenkrais maintained that most people use only 5 percent of the options available. Like other proponents of movement re-education, Feldenkrais believed that our habits of movement are established in early childhood.

Through repetition, these patterns become fixed in our central nervous system, created not only by physical factors but psychological ones as well. A child who is surrounded by joy and laughter will develop habits that are different from a child whose environment is full of fear and anger.

These unconscious patterns need not be permanent, however. Feldenkrais believed that it was possible to re-educate the central nervous system to recognize other possibilities for movement and choose those that are more efficient and free. He felt that the body has an intuitive sense that allows it to recognize more appropriate movement, if only it is given the chance to learn that movement. Poor habits can be broken even by experiencing better habits just once, so great is the power of the unconscious mind to learn what is right.

Feldenkrais believed that people are aware of the front and

upper parts of their bodies, but not the back or legs. His goal was for students to achieve a total body awareness that would allow them to move with a sense of freedom that tapped into their full potential. To that end, Feldenkrais developed a system of several thousand exercises that stimulated the muscles and brain and helped them learn better ways to move.

Feldenkrais brought his method to this country in the early 1970s with the help of the Esalen Institute—a patron to many forerunners of body-work. In 1977, he established the Feldenkrais Guild in San Francisco, which is the training organization for teachers of the Feldenkrais Method.

WHAT IT IS

The thing that makes the Feldenkrais Method different from other types of movement re-education is its focus on gently prying habits of move-ment from our unconscious mind and bringing them into conscious awareness. There are two main forms of the Felden-krais Method: "awareness through movement" and "func-tional integration."

Awareness through movement is offered in a series of group lessons. The focus is on mak-ing students aware of how they move through very slow, de-tailed exploration of certain individual movements, such as bending or reaching. Often classes are offered to address specific issues, such as tem-poromandibular joint pain, how to sit better, or enhancing athletic performance. Teachers also use verbal instructions and guided imagery to lead students through very small, precise movements, such as raising their leg. The goal is to make students aware of how to make fine adjustments that use their full potential.

Functional integration offers individual instruction that combines oral instruction with gentle touch. The student lies fully clothed on a padded table while the teacher uses his hands to observe movement patterns and suggest alternatives. Un-like chiropractic or massage, the teacher does not manipulate the body. Instead, he gently guides the student through a series of precise movements that are aimed at making him aware of more efficient ways to move. Rather than working with bones or soft tissue, the Feldenkrais teacher works with the nervous system, reprogram-ming it to adopt new ways of moving.

USES

The Feldenkrais Method can help alleviate a variety of disorders, but the focus is on learning, not curing. The teacher helps students understand how their movements may exacerbate the condition, then teaches them to move in ways that are more comfortable and can alleviate physical stress.

Though Feldenkrais was famous for his work with neuromuscular disorders, studies of long-term benefits have not been done. Practitioners have found it to benefit:

* low-back pain
* temporomandibular disorder (TMD)
* headaches
* neck and shoulder pain
* arthritis
* muscular disorders

The Feldenkrais Method also can decrease pain and improve range of motion in stroke and accident victims. Those who engage in strenuous physical activity, including athletes, dancers, and musicians, often find the method beneficial. Finally, it may be helpful to anyone who simply wants to reduce physical tension and feel a greater sense of fluidity and grace of movement.

WHO PERFORMS IT

The Feldenkrais Guild has trained and certified about 2,500 practitioners, many of them in Israel and Europe. The Feldenkrais program includes instruction and hands-on work. After completing half the training program, a practitioner is allowed to teach awareness-through-movement classes.

HELLERWORK

A student of Ida Rolf, Joseph Heller eventually branched out and developed his own form of touch therapy. Hellerwork focuses on helping people make connections between what is happening in their life and how that affects their body. The goal is to break free of chronic patterns of mental and physical tension.

HISTORY

Joseph Heller began his career in the early 1960s with a degree in mathematics from the California Institute of Technology (Cal Tech). He spent a decade working as an aerospace engineer, analyzing the effects of gravity and stress on space rockets. Seeking relief from the demands of his high-stress job, Heller became interested in encounter groups and manipulative therapies in the late 1960s and early 1970s.

Eventually, he met Ida Rolf and studied under her. He became a certified Rolfer (see Rolfing, page 94) and eventually was elected the first president of the Rolf Institute. While at the Rolf Institute, Heller met Judith Aston, a protégée of Rolf who was developing her own ideas about movement re-education (see Aston-Patterning, page 41).

As he studied and practiced bodywork, Heller realized that clients talked about certain subjects when he touched certain parts of the body. He developed strongly held views that the body stores emotions and attitudes and that the psychological profoundly affects the physical. Eventually, in the late 1970s, Heller broke away from the Rolf Institute, arguing that restructuring the body through manipulation alone would not prove to have lasting effects.

The approach Heller developed combines deep-tissue manipulation with exercises that help clients perform everyday movements such as sitting and standing without physical stress. (Rolfing eventually incorporated movement re-education exercises too.) Hellerwork also emphasizes mind/body techniques designed to release emotional stress and trauma.

WHAT IT IS

Hellerwork is a program of 11 sessions, each lasting 90 minutes, each with a different focus. It is suggested that you have one session a week, but some people schedule one session a month, while others do the whole program in just a few weeks. In the 11 sessions you will focus on such topics as inspiration, control, gut feelings, and reaching out (see box, page, 59).

According to Heller, there are three primary causes of stress in the body: physical trauma, emotional trauma, and misuse. Hellerwork addresses each of these causes and is meant to realign the body, release chronic tension, and create a more relaxed state of being.

Deep-tissue massage focuses on releasing tightness in the fascia—the connective tissue that envelops all the muscles and joins them to the bones. Eradicating fascial tension brings the body into better vertical alignment.

Movement re-education makes patients aware of how they use their bodies to perform daily activities. Clients typically are videotaped, then shown new ways to sit, stand, walk, and move. The practitioner uses suggestion and visualization to help patients achieve greater alignment and fluidity.

Finally, guided verbal dialogue allows the practitioner and patient to explore emotions triggered by the bodywork. The dialogue focuses on a different theme each session.

USES

Hellerwork is not aimed at curing illness but rather releasing chronic physical and emotional stress and developing more fluid patterns of movement. Controlled research on Hellerwork has not been conducted, but practitioners have found that it benefits a variety of conditions, including:

* stress
* low energy and fatigue
* poor posture
* chronic muscular pain, particularly in the neck, shoulders, and back
* respiratory problems
* sports injuries

WHO PERFORMS IT

Hellerwork, Inc., trains practitioners all over the world. The format varies, but the curriculum is the same for each train-

THE HELLERWORK SERIES

The Hellerwork program comprises 11 sessions of 90 minutes each. Each session has a different theme, and the bodywork, movement re-education, and guided verbal dialogue of a particular session focuses on that theme.

❋ *Inspiration:* Designed to open up the breathing and align the rib cage over the pelvis. Patients are asked to pay attention to things that inspire or depress them and how those things affect their breathing.

❋ *Standing on Your Own Two Feet:* Aligns the legs and redistributes body weight. Patients think about issues of security and how stable they are financially, emotionally, and interpersonally.

❋ *Reaching Out:* Releases tension in the shoulders, arms, and sides. Patients examine what happens when they don't pursue what they want out of life.

❋ *Control and Surrender:* Focuses on releasing tension in the legs and pelvic floor. Patients consider what things they want to dominate and what they want to surrender to.

❋ *The Guts:* Elongates the front of the body's core. Patients notice gut feelings.

❋ *Holding Back:* Lengthens the back of the body's core. Clients pay attention to what happens when they practice restraint.

❋ *Losing Your Head:* Releases tension in the head, neck, and face. Patients think about excessive analytic tendencies.

❋ *The Feminine:* Alleviates rotations in the legs, feet, and pelvis. Clients ponder the role the feminine principle plays in their lives.

❋ *The Masculine:* Releases rotations in the arms, shoulders, rib cage, and neck. Clients concentrate on easily performing penetrating actions with their upper torso.

❋ *Integration:* Works on increasing joint movement. Clients pay attention to integrity and issues of separation.

❋ *Coming Out:* Resolves any outstanding physical and emotional issues.

ing. A list of trained practitioners is available from Hellerwork, Inc. (see Appendix, page 245). The rates charged for the 11 sessions vary, but the normal range is between $60 and $120 depending on your location and need.

INFANT MASSAGE

Touch is such an essential human need that babies will waste away without it. Performing infant massage helps parents build strong bonds with their babies, and it also relaxes both parent and child.

HISTORY

Baby massage is an ancient tradition in many cultures throughout the world. In rural India, for instance, children receive massages every day from infancy through toddlerhood. Traditionally, baby massage there is performed with a dough ball dipped in oil for the first few weeks, to clean the child and stimulate circulation. Then it is done with the hands, using different types of vegetable oil that vary with the season. Particular attention is given to stroking the spine, to help give it strength to support the body.

Baby massage was introduced to this country in the early 1970s by Vimala Schneider McClure, a young American woman who discovered the practice while working in an orphanage in India. After returning to the United States, she continued to research the subject and eventually developed a curriculum for parent-child classes. Her book *Infant Massage: A Handbook for Loving Parents* received an enthusiastic response when it was published in 1977, and she went on to found the International Association of Infant Massage, which certifies instructors who teach infant-massage classes across the country.

WHAT IT IS

Infant massage is basically a modified form of Swedish massage. The giver—usually a parent—uses gentle stroking, squeezing, and pressure-point techniques to provide the baby with loving, nurturing contact. Massage is usually performed beginning a few weeks after birth, continuing through toddlerhood. Many babies have a time during the day when they tend to be fussy; if given an hour before this time, massage can help soothe babies and reduce fussiness.

A baby massage typically begins with the legs, because this is the least vulnerable part of a baby's body and helps them adjust to being massaged. Stroking the bottom of the foot with firm thumb pressure helps stimulate nerve endings, just like reflexology massage, and firm, milking strokes from ankle to hip is beneficial for babies with poor muscle tone.

Strokes on the abdomen help tone the digestive system and can ease gas and constipation. Strokes on the chest, arms, and face follow, then the baby is turned over for a back massage. Stroking firmly with a swooping motion from the neck to the buttocks can thoroughly relax and calm a baby.

USES

Infant massage has numerous benefits. Research has found that massage of premature babies helps them gain weight faster and shortens their hospital stay. Massage also:

* improves bonding between parent and child
* makes babies more easily soothed
* prompts the baby's body to release endorphins, natural painkillers that produce a sense of well being
* lowers levels of stress hormones
* promotes deeper sleep
* increases alertness and responsiveness while awake
* reduces episodes of apnea, or cessation of breathing, which can cause sudden infant death syndrome (SIDS)
* alleviates colic and gas
* enhances the immune-system functioning

Infant massage also has benefits for the parents who perform it. Their parenting skills and confidence in their skills are increased. Fathers, who often don't get to spend as much time nurturing babies, may especially enjoy the chance for close, one-on-one contact, and it can be an excellent way for either parent to reconnect with a child after being away at work all day. And, nursing mothers who perform massage experi-

EASING COLIC

A bout of colic can make a baby's first few weeks of life miserable for both her and her parents. Infant massage can help alleviate colic, as well as gas and constipation.

* First, use a firm, scooping motion to sweep the right hand from the top of the abdomen to the bottom, followed immediately by the left hand. Repeat several times.
* Gently push the knees to the belly and hold for about half a minute.
* Using one hand, stroke firmly and slowly in a clockwise circle on the abdomen. Repeat several times.
* Gently push the knees to the belly and hold for about half a minute. Repeat this sequence three times, several times a day. It may take a few days before you notice the colic abating.

ence an increase in levels of prolactin, a hormone that stimulates milk production.

WHO PERFORMS IT

The International Association of Infant Massage certifies instructors of infant massage, who teach classes for parents and caregivers across the country. A large number of massage therapists have also taken training in infant massage.

Current research

The Touch Research Institute in Miami, Fla., is a pioneer in studying the effects of touch on a wide variety of health problems. The Institute conducted the landmark research that found premature babies who were massaged three times a day gained 47 percent more weight than the non-massaged babies—even though both groups had the same calorie intake. The researchers found that massage stimulated the infants' brains to release more insulin, which helped the babies' bodies use their food more efficiently.

Currently, the Touch Research Institute is exploring the benefits of touch for:

* newborns of cocaine-addicted mothers
* HIV-exposed newborns
* infants of depressed mothers
* infant sleep disorders
* infants with cancer

JIN SHIN DO

Translated as "the way of the compassionate spirit,"
Jin Shin Do is a type of acupressure aimed at releasing
physical and emotional tension.

HISTORY

Technically known as Jin Shin Do Bodymind Acupressure, this healing modality was developed by psychotherapist and massage therapist Iona Marsaa Teeguarden, who studied acupuncture and acupressure under masters in the United States and Japan and founded the Jin Shin Do Foundation in 1982. With her training in psychotherapy, Teeguarden saw emotions as essentially a positive force guiding people to self-awareness. If emotions become blocked, however, they create physical tension and negative states of functioning. Jin Shin Do was created as both a professional and self-help technique for enhancing personal growth.

WHAT IT IS

Like acupressure, Jin Shin Do is based on the Chinese concept of qi, the vital life force that animates all living beings. This life force flows throughout the body along 12 main channels, called meridians, each

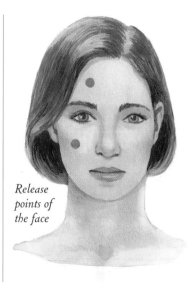

Release points of the face

associated with a particular organ. Disease is the result of either blocked or weak qi.

Unlike other types of acupressure, Jin Shin Do is the only one that uses what are called "strange flows," which are part of the meridian system. These are channels that connect with and monitor the flow of qi in the 12 main meridians; they collect and release energy. Traditionally, in Chinese medicine, these are believed to be holding places for the body's essence and aren't often used. In Jin Shin Do, however, they are viewed as important self-regulating devices—rather like reservoirs and dams—and are used frequently.

Practitioners can help balance the flow of qi by applying pressure to 45 main release points among the hundreds of acupoints located along the meridians. (The layperson technique uses 30 primary points.) The practitioner uses finger pressure on local points for a minute or two while also applying pressure to distal points, to improve the release of tension.

Applying the right type of pressure is essential and depends on whether the point is in a yin part of the body or a yang part. In areas of yin—which, in Chinese medicine, represents female energy—the practitioner's arm sinks into the point. In areas that are yang—or associated with male energy—stronger pressure can be used, with the practitioner leaning into the point.

USES

Jin Shin Do has not been studied in controlled trials, but presumably findings on acupuncture and acupressure have implications for its benefits. Practitioners say it is helpful for headaches, insomnia, back pain, stress, fatigue, and negative emotional states.

WHO PERFORMS IT

Training in Jin Shin Do is offered to professionals who are licensed or certified in some sort of healing discipline. After completing the required coursework and practice hours, practitioners may become registered through the Jin Shin Do Foundation.

JIN SHIN JYUTSU

This type of bodywork doesn't involve manipulation of soft tissue but rather gentle laying-on of hands that is aimed at balancing the flow of energy in the body.

HISTORY

Jin Shin Jyutsu is believed to be an ancient art that dates back before the birth of Buddha. For many centuries the tradition was handed down orally in Tibet and China before making its way to Japan. The techniques eventually disappeared until they were revived in the 1900s by the Japanese philosopher Jiro Murai.

Diagnosed with a terminal illness while in his 20s, Murai retreated to his family's cabin in the mountains to die. He told his family to come to the cabin after 7 days. During his time of solitude, Murai meditated and practiced healing hand poses he had learned from observing the actions of various sages. For 6 days, Murai felt himself become colder and colder and was sure he was about to die. On the seventh day, however, he recovered and vowed to spend his life learning and teaching Jin Shin Jyutsu.

The technique was brought to the United States in the late 1970s by Mary Burmeister, who met Murai when she went to Japan in the 1940s to study the language. She spent more than a decade studying under Murai before she began teaching Jin Shin Jyutsu in this country.

WHAT IT IS

As with other Eastern forms of healing, Jin Shin Jyutsu holds that there is a vital life energy, called qi, that flows throughout the body along various energy channels. Physical, emotional, or mental disorders are signs that this energy has become blocked in any of 26 different points called safety energy locks.

HANDY SELF-CARE TIPS

You don't have to find a Jin Shin Jyutsu practitioner to take advantage of its benefits; it's also meant to be a powerful self-help tool. According to Jin Shin Jyutsu principles, each finger is associated with various emotional states. By holding a particular finger for a few minutes until a quiet, rhythmic pulse is felt, you can harmonize these different states. Here's a guide:

❋ The thumb is associated with worry.
❋ The index finger is associated with fear.
❋ The middle finger is associated with anger.
❋ The ring finger is associated with sadness.
❋ The little finger is associated with pretense.

To help clear the blockages and allow qi to flow freely, a practitioner places her hands in proscribed positions on the safety energy locks. The practitioner does not give her own energy to the receiver but serves as a conduit through which universal energy flows. This universal energy acts to release the patient's energy from blocked points, which restores harmony and stimulates the body to heal itself.

USES

Clinical research of Jin Shin Jyutsu has not been performed.

Practitioners emphasize that it is not meant to heal or cure any illness but instead is a tool for rebalancing energy and allowing the body to heal itself of physical, emotional, or mental distress.

WHO PERFORMS IT

Mary Burmeister has authored several books aimed at teaching laypeople self-help Jin Shin Jyutsu. Seminars for practitioners are offered throughout the United States by the Jin Shin Jyutsu Center. (For more information, see Appendix, page 246.)

MANUAL LYMPH DRAINAGE

The lymphatic system is essential to protecting against disease and infection. Among other functions, it filters bacteria, viruses, water, and other impurities from the blood; it carries white blood cells; and it produces antibodies. Unlike the circulatory system, which is driven by the heart, the lymphatic system does not have its own internal pump. Massage is one way to enhance its flow.

HISTORY

Manual lymph drainage is a massage technique developed in the 1930s by husband and wife massage therapists Dr. Emil Vodder and his wife, Astrid. The Vodders practiced on the French Riviera, where a

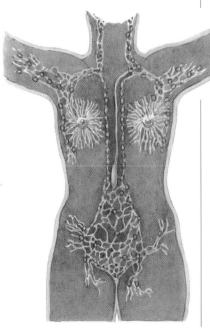

great many of their clients were vacationing Britons who suffered from chronic colds, sinusitis, and other respiratory ailments, due to the cold, damp weather back home.

Dr. Vodder noticed that the majority of these patients had swollen lymph nodes and theorized that blockage there could be the cause of their chronic infections. Although conventional wisdom suggested that the lymphatic system not be worked on directly, the Vodders began massaging the swollen lymph nodes anyway, and their patients' illnesses disappeared.

The Vodders spent a number of years in Paris perfecting their technique, which they called Dr. Vodder's manual lymph drainage. World War II prompted them to return to their native Denmark, where they established the Manual Lymphatic Drainage Institute—a training center in Copenhagen. They eventually handed their duties over to two students, who in the 1970s founded the Dr. Vodder School in Walchsee, Austria.

Manual lymph drainage eventually spread throughout Europe, and today it is one of the most prescribed physical therapies in Germany. It was introduced to the United States and Canada in the 1980s and is now taught in many massage schools.

WHAT IT IS

Manual lymph drainage uses slow, repetitive strokes to enhance circulation in the lymphatic system, which is responsible for removing excess water, waste, and toxins from the connective tissue that surrounds all the cells in the body. Lymph is the clear or milky fluid that runs through a system of ducts outside the bloodstream and is filtered by lymph nodes located throughout the system.

The practitioner always strokes in the same direction the muscle fiber runs to help push along the lymph. The touch is fairly gentle, because much of the lymph lies in the top layers of tissue, rather than deeper in the body.

There are 5 primary strokes, which are performed in a proscribed pattern:

* stationary circles
* moving thumb circles
* pumping
* scooping
* rotary

The rhythmic action of the strokes increases the absorption of lymph from connective tissue into the lymph system. It also helps the circulatory system absorb waste from the body's tissues and carry it away.

USES

Research has shown that manual lymph drainage is very effective for reducing edema—a condition in which the body's tissues contain an excess amount of fluid, leading to swelling. This therapy is of particular benefit in lymphedema, a common type of edema in which the circulation of the lymphatic system is impaired. Lymphedema can occur for a variety of reasons. A person may be born with it, for instance, or may develop it when lymph nodes are surgically removed because they are

THE LYMPHATIC SYSTEM

If you've ever had red, swollen tonsils, you've seen firsthand the effects of an impaired lymphatic system. Here's a quick guide to understanding the system:

❋ Lymph is a clear fluid that flows through lymph vessels and carries white blood cells. It must fight gravity to do its job, because much of the time it flows from the bottom of the body up toward the heart.

❋ More than 600 bean-size lymph nodes are scattered throughout the body. These act like a cleanup crew, filtering toxins and waste from the lymph and producing antibodies to fight disease. They kick into high gear during serious illness: They're capable of manufacturing 2,000 antibodies per second.

❋ Lymph glands are manufacturing and processing centers for various components of the immune system, such as lymphocytes and T cells. Lymph glands include the spleen, thymus gland, and tonsils.

cancerous, after a mastectomy, for example.

Among other benefits, manual lymph drainage:

❋ enhances immunity
❋ promotes post-surgical or post-traumatic healing by carrying away waste products
❋ reduces chronic inflammation
❋ reduces stagnation, or stasis, of lymph flow
❋ induces relaxation

WHO PERFORMS IT

The Dr. Vodder School in Walchsee, Austria, certifies practitioners who complete its intensive four-week course and pass an examination. It is estimated that there are about 250 certified therapists in North America. Also, many massage schools teach manual lymph drainage, so ask your practitioner about his training in the technique.

MEDICAL MASSAGE

America is the only industrialized nation where massage isn't an official part of the health care system. In Germany and throughout the former Soviet Union and China, every major hospital has a massage therapy department. Massage also is found in medical settings in India and Japan. Slowly, though, the medical establishment in North America is beginning to recognize the value of massage.

HISTORY

Therapeutic massage was introduced to the United States in the 1850s by physicians George and Charles Taylor. The two brothers studied massage in Sweden and England, then returned home to New York and began using it in their practice. In the 1870s, two Swedes were responsible for opening the first U.S. massage therapy clinics— one in Boston and one in Washington, D.C. The clinic in the capitol attracted a number of famous clients, including Presidents Benjamin Harrison and Ulysses S. Grant.

In the early 1900s, the medical system in this country focused increasingly on technology-based therapies, such as drugs and surgery. Time-pressed because they had so many patients as a result of World War I, physicians became less interested in hands-on healing and handed over massage duties to nurses and assistants. Eventually, these practitioners also lost interest in massage in favor of mechanical and electrical apparatuses, and it was left to a small number of therapists to continue the practice until the late 1960s, when natural medicine slowly began to experience a revival. The Swedish Institute in New York City became the first massage school to open a medical massage clinic; patients must have a doctor's referral to be treated there.

Today, therapeutic massage is extremely popular with the general public, and it can be found in an increasing number of medical settings, though it still is usually not practiced by physicians. Rather, massage therapists are employed to provide care for patients; massage lessens their pain and helps speed healing. Also, some physicians are willing to refer patients to massage therapists for treatment of specific health conditions. Massage therapy is also used outside of medical settings and is used for stress management, relaxation, and reduction of muscle tension.

WHAT IT IS

Medical massage is simply therapeutic massage that is focused on a particular health issue. Typically, medical massage uses various techniques of Swedish massage to target a medically diagnosed condition:

❋ *Effleurage*, which means "touching lightly," is a smooth, gliding stroke that is done in the direction of the heart to stimulate circulation of blood and lymph. This stroke is especially beneficial in cases of inflammation, because it helps remove waste products and excess fluid.

❋ *Petrissage*, or kneading, lifts muscles away from bone, then rolls and kneads them, like bread dough. Like effleurage, petrissage stimulates circulation of blood and lymph, and also helps prevent muscle atrophy.

❋ *Friction*, or rubbing, is the deepest of the strokes. It involves deep circular or transverse strokes that cause layers of tissue to rub against one another. The goal of friction is to break down adhesions and make muscles and joints more supple. Friction is especially useful for treating muscle spasms and easing stiffness in the joints.

❋ *Tapotment*, or tapping, is also known as percussion or pounding. Typically using the edge of her hands, the therapist strikes the patient's body with rapid, alternating blows. The effects of percussion vary according to the length of time the stroke is applied. When administered for less than 10 seconds, it is stimulating and causes tissue contraction, which can help remove blood from an area. When applied for a longer period, of up to a minute, it helps flush an area with blood. More than 60 seconds of tapotment fatigues the muscles, which can be beneficial for those that are cramped or in spasm.

❋ *Vibration*, or shaking, is like tapotment in that it can be either stimulating or relaxing, depending on how long it is performed. The practitioner uses shaking movements with the hands or fingers. It is especially beneficial for stimulating nerve activity.

USES

Medical massage is typically performed on the advice of a physician for any number of conditions:

* low-back pain
* fibromyalgia
* tendinitis
* sciatica
* repetitive stress disorders, such as carpal tunnel syndrome
* temporomandibular disorder (TMD)
* sprains and strains
* irritable bowel syndrome and other digestive disorders

WHO PERFORMS IT

Currently, it is estimated that there are as many as 150,000 massage therapists in the United States. Massage therapists are licensed in 25 states and the District of Columbia. In the remaining states, local government bodies may regulate the practice generally. In addition, there is a national board that certifies practitioners: the National Certification Board for Therapeutic Massage and Bodywork (NCBTMB).

Because licensing is not available to all practitioners, you may want to ask whether a therapist is affiliated with an organization such as the American Massage Therapy Association (AMTA), which has stringent guidelines for membership, including, at a minimum, completion of an accredited massage therapy program. AMTA has about 30,000 members in more than 20 countries and is massage therapy's largest and oldest professional organization.

MYOFASCIAL RELEASE

Myofascial release is a technique that frees muscles
from the grip of overly tense fascia, the connective
tissue that covers virtually all parts of the body,
including muscles, bones, nerves, and organs.

HISTORY

Myofascial release was developed by John Barnes, a physical therapist, in the 1960s and '70s. As a teenager, Barnes had a weightlifting accident that crushed one of the disks in his lower back. He opted for spinal-fusion surgery, which proved to be beneficial, though he still experienced pain. As an adult, Barnes re-injured himself when he stumbled into a gopher hole on a backpacking trip. By this time, he had become a physical therapist, and he decided to try self-help massage techniques.

Trained in soft-tissue mobilization, Barnes found that when working on himself, he had to adapt these methods and work more gently on the tissue, simply holding pressure for extended periods of time—which proved to be key to his success. Eventually, Barnes took a seminar on connective tissue and realized that he had intuitively been working on releasing restrictions in his fascia, which alleviated much of his pain.

Barnes began further developing myofascial release after he treated a patient with severe back and neck pain. Not having time to work on both areas, he used his techniques on just on her lower back. He was stunned when, after the session, the patient had regained most of the range of motion in her neck, driving home the point that restriction in one part of the fascia can have affects in remote parts of the body. Today, Barnes lectures all over the world, and a growing number of physical therapists are incorporating his techniques in their work.

WHAT IT IS

Fascia is a continuous sheet of connective tissue that is woven among all the cells of the body. There are two types of fibers that make up the fascia: collagenous fibers that are very tough and have little stretchability and elastic fibers that are stretchable. Fascia covers all the tissues and organs, giving the body form; if every part of a human but the fascia were removed—all the muscles, bones, and organs—the body would still retain its shape.

Injury, inflammation, and bad posture are just some of the factors that can cause abnormal pressure on the fascia. Because fascia is interconnected and pervades the entire body, tension in one part of the fascia can cause problems in other, seemingly unrelated areas. To release tension in the fascia, practitioners use steady, fairly gentle hand pressure to stretch the tissue, holding it until the tissue relaxes. The process is repeated until no further stretching is possible.

Gentle touch is essential to myofascial release. While muscle tissue responds to firm pressure, the collagenous fibers of fascia are extremely tough and resistant to stretching.

They will, however, begin to loosen under mild pressure that is sustained—much like taffy stretches with small, steady pressure.

Chronic conditions may require several months of treatment to eradicate fascial restrictions. Practitioners often give range of motion and stretching exercises to help patients maintain progress between sessions.

USES

Though clinical studies of myofascial release have not been done, practitioners say it is beneficial for nearly any condition involving muscle tightness, including back, neck, and jaw pain, and stress.

WHO PERFORMS IT

Practitioners receive training in myofascial release from seminars offered across the country. For the most part, myofascial release tends to be used by massage therapists, chiropractors, and physical therapists.

ON-SITE MASSAGE

These days, on-the-job demands seem to be greater than ever. The era of corporate downsizing has meant that fewer people are left to do more work. The result is employees who suffer from stress, headaches, exhaustion, and even lowered resistance to illness. On-site massage is a quick way to ease workplace stress and tension.

HISTORY

On-site massage, also known as seated massage, was developed in the early 1980s by oriental-massage therapist David Palmer, owner of a massage school. Looking for a way to create work for his graduates, he began developing the idea of seated massage. Within a few years, he created the first massage chair, a portable, lightweight padded chair that slopes forward and has a face cradle. With the chair, Palmer taught techniques and business strategies for chair massage.

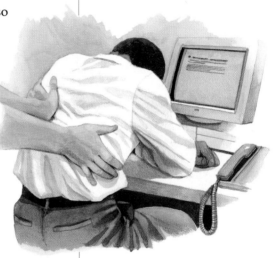

Today, on-site massage is one of the fastest-growing fields of massage therapy. Companies that have used the service of on-site practitioners include Reebok, American Express, AT&T, and Merrill Lynch. Seated massage isn't offered only in the workplace either; you'll also find it at airports, convention centers, shopping malls, even on street corners.

WHAT IT IS

On-site seated massage is typically of shorter duration than table massage—usually

THE COST OF STRESS

Stress takes a huge toll in the workplace:

✻ 85 percent of employee accidents are stress-related.

✻ Each year, stress accounts for $26 billion in medical and disability payments.

✻ Stress keeps about one million people a day from going to work.

✻ Stress leads one-third of American workers to consider quitting their jobs.

around 15 to 30 minutes. The client remains clothed and no oil is used. The practitioner focuses on the areas where people tend to hold their stress: the neck, back, and shoulders. In some cases, the practitioner may also massage the scalp, arms, and legs. In keeping with Palmer's specialty in oriental massage, seated massage tends to rely on shiatsu techniques.

USES

On-site massage focuses on reducing stress and its effects. Among other benefits, it:

✻ reduces muscle tension and pain

✻ calms the nervous system and increases circulation

✻ helps employees identify and release tension on their own

One recent study found that a 15-minute massage significantly boosted job performance. Compared with workers who spent the same amount of time simply taking a break, the employees who received massage completed math problems in half the time with half the errors. After a month of regular treatment, their anxiety levels were markedly reduced.

WHO PERFORMS IT

Many massage schools educate students in seated massage, and David Palmer alone has trained several thousand therapists in the technique. Unfortunately, however, on-site massage is not legal in all municipalities. Many places outlawed the practice years ago as a way to control "massage parlors" that were fronts for prostitution. Massage therapists are working to change these laws.

OSTEOPATHIC MEDICINE

Osteopathic medicine can be a good place to start an exploration of complementary medicine because it combines conventional and complementary approaches. Osteopathic physicians are qualified to provide the full range of medical services a conventional medical doctor, or M.D., uses—such as prescribing drugs and performing surgery—but they're trained to take a holistic approach that favors using noninvasive, hands-on techniques first.

HISTORY

Osteopathic medicine was founded by a 19th-century surgeon named Andrew Taylor Still. After losing three children to the meningitis epidemic of 1864, Still became a vocal critic of Western medicine, criticizing it for what he believed were ineffective and, at times, even harmful methods of treatment.

Still believed that the body has an innate self-healing power. Rather than attacking symptoms with drugs and invasive medical techniques, he thought physicians needed to look for the underlying cause of illness, then encourage the body's own innate ability to solve the problem itself. Still viewed patients as whole people, with each part interdependent on all the others. The medical system

he developed was based on this idea of unity, and he identified the musculoskeletal system as being key to overall health.

According to Still, human touch was vital to establishing patient confidence in a doctor, and he emphasized using the hands to help diagnose and treat injury and illness. Physical manipulation became the underpinning of his technique. He also incorporated physical exercise and advice on diet and lifestyle factors. Still pioneered the concept of "wellness" that has become popular only in recent years.

In the early part of this century, osteopathic physicians fought many legal battles against M.D.s who tried to prohibit them from practicing. By the 1920s the profession had gained a fair amount of credibility, as nearly all states implemented regulations governing the practice of osteopathic medicine.

Today, the federal government and the American Medical Association recognize doctors of osteopathy, or D.O.s, as being equal to M.D.s. The profession received an image boost in 1996 when, for the first time, an osteopathic physician became surgeon general of the U.S. Army. That year another D.O. was named director of emergency medicine for the Olympic Village at the games in Atlanta.

as primary care family doctors, often in small towns that tend to be medically underserved.

WHAT IT IS

While conventional medical students tend to choose a specialty by their second or third year of school, osteopathic physicians are trained to be generalists first and specialists second. Although some do go on to specialize after receiving their degree, a great many osteopathic physicians practice

Osteopathic medicine puts particular emphasis on keenly using the senses when treating patients, particularly the senses of sight and touch. A D.O. visually examines the patient's body for asymmetry, then palpates (feels) the patient's body with his hands. The doctor may also have the patient perform range of motion exercises and palpate each area as it's being exercised, looking for abnormalities in soft tissues, such as contraction or swelling. Such changes offer important clues to health; one osteopathic research study, for example, found clear changes in the

The Healing Power of Touch

Osteopathic Approaches

Osteopathic physicians employ a variety of techniques to perform physical manipulation and help the body restore its equilibrium. Here are some of the most used:

※ Strain-Counterstrain Therapy alleviates tenderness and pain caused by trigger points, which are hypersensitive areas that refer pain to another part of the body. A trigger point in the back, for instance, may cause a feeling of pain near the elbow. Using strain-counterstrain, the doctor moves the body into a position that relieves the referred pain, then holds it. When the body is moved back to its original position and the trigger point is stimulated, the referred pain is gone.

※ Cranial techniques, also called craniosacral therapy, uses very gentle manipulation to release tension and dysfunction in the structure and fluid of the craniosacral system (see pages 51–53).

※ Lymphatic drainage involves rhythmically applying pressure to the upper chest to stimulate circulation of lymph, the fluid that carries white blood cells and is important to immunity (see pages 67–69).

※ The soft-tissue technique is used mainly around the spine and relies on stretching and deep pressure to relax muscles and increase circulation.

※ Myofascial release focuses on alleviating restrictions in the fascia, the connective tissue that surrounds all the muscles and organs in the body (see pages 73–74).

※ Thrust technique is a thrusting motion that restores range of motion to joints.

※ In the muscle-energy technique, the physician uses counterforce as the patient tenses and releases specific muscles. The goal is to relax the muscles.

upper back that were related to heart disease.

A fundamental philosophy of osteopathic medicine is that impairment in any part of the musculoskeletal system—the nerves, muscles, and bones—affects the rest of the body. To stimulate the body's self-healing abilities, osteopathic physicians rely on physical manipulation to correct structural problems. The focus of manipulation is different from chiropractic, which concentrates on misaligned joints; osteopaths tends to use soft-tissue treatment to relax muscles and restore joint mobility.

USES

Because they're licensed in the full scope of practice, osteopathic physicians can benefit just about any condition for which you would visit an M.D., including infection, injury, and pain. Because of their expertise in musculoskeletal issues and their training in physical manipulation, however, D.O.s are particularly well suited to treat conditions such as:

* back pain—One study that compared osteopathic manipulation with massage for low-back pain found osteopathic treatment provided greater relief.
* carpal tunnel syndrome—Research has shown that osteopathic techniques, particularly myofascial release, improve various symptoms and reduce the need for surgery.
* pediatric neurologic dysfunction—One study showed that young children with neurologic impairments improved significantly after a series of osteopathic treatments.

WHO PERFORMS IT

There are more than 40,000 osteopathic physicians in this country, representing around 6 percent of the total physicians in the United States. Osteopathic physicians have a medical education as thorough as that of M.D.s. They receive their D.O. degree after four years of study, then work at a one-year internship. A two- to six-year residency may follow if the physician wants to specialize.

Doctors of osteopathy are licensed to render complete medical care in all 50 states and the District of Columbia. They can diagnose medical conditions, prescribe medication, and perform surgery. Many D.O.s specialize in various branches of medicine, including psychiatry, obstetrics, and geriatrics.

Keep in mind that although osteopathic physicians are trained in physical manipulation, only about 5 percent actually use it in their practice. If you want someone skilled in this type of treatment, be sure to ask whether he or she uses it; you may want to look for a practitioner with continuing education credits or teaching experience in manipulation.

PHYSICAL THERAPY

Physical therapy has always been a hands-on profession, dedicated to restoring physical function in patients with a wide variety of ailments, from birth defects to sports injuries. However, some practitioners are going beyond the traditional techniques of their trade, such as joint mobilization and ultrasound, to incorporate more alternative touch therapies, such as acupressure, craniosacral therapy, and the Alexander Technique.

HISTORY

The therapeutic techniques used by modern-day physical therapists in many cases date back to ancient times. Heat therapy came from the Egyptians, who worshiped the healing power of the sun. Early Greek and Roman cultures also used heat therapy, and the Romans and Chinese made use of hydrotherapy, or healing with water. Middle Eastern doctors used exercise therapeutically during the Dark Ages, and the British were using massage as early as the 1500s.

The present-day practice of physical therapy originated during World War I. In need of practitioners who could rehabilitate wounded soldiers, the U.S. Surgeon General's Office created the Division of Special Hospitals and Reconstruction. The division hired 2,000 "reconstruction aides," who worked in hospitals and used muscle re-education, hydrotherapy, electrical stimulation, corrective exercises, and massage to treat patients.

In 1921, a group of women reconstruction aides formed the American Women's Physical Therapeutic Association. By the end of the 1930s, men were permitted to join and the name was changed to the American Physiotherapy Association; the group boasted around 1,000 members.

The need for physical therapists escalated with World War II and the polio epidemic of the 1940s and 1950s, and the ranks of physical therapists swelled eightfold. Adversity once again stimulated growth of the profession in the 1960s, when prosthetics and orthotics were needed for babies born to mothers who had taken thalidomide—an anti-morning-sickness drug that caused physical deformities.

The documented benefits of physical therapy for nearly any kind of physical problem has led to tremendous growth of the field during the past two decades. Although there currently are more than 120,000 physical therapists in the United States, there is still a shortage of practitioners to meet demand.

WHAT IT IS

Physical therapists are qualified to evaluate and treat problems related to physical function. The goal is to help patients regain as much normal physical function as quickly as possible. Treatments are meant to reduce swelling, relieve pain, increase strength and range of motion, and prevent injury. Physical therapists generally employ mechanical and electrical equipment a great deal in their work. In some cases, physical therapists must help patients relearn how to perform the most basic tasks of everyday living, such as dressing or bathing.

Physical therapists have a wide variety of modalities at their disposal, including:

- corrective exercises
- joint mobilization
- cardiovascular endurance training
- relaxation exercises
- biofeedback
- electrical stimulation
- hydrotherapy
- traction
- heat
- ultrasound
- ice therapy
- laser therapy
- manipulation
- therapeutic massage

In addition, some therapists are incorporating more alternative approaches, including acupressure, craniosacral therapy, the Alexander Technique, the Feldenkrais Method, and Therapeutic Touch. These techniques are not generally included in the academic program in physical therapy school; for the most part, practitioners study and become certified in them on their own.

Physical therapy also focuses on teaching patients how to continue their progress at home. Not only does the therapist often prescribe a continuing exercise program for the patient, but she may

The Healing Power of Touch

also include instruction on wellness and safety. Physical therapists educate patients about the importance of fitness by designing conditioning programs for individuals, and they teach people how to avoid injury in a variety of situations.

USES

Many physical therapists work in hospitals, but the majority work in private practice or places like clinics, physical-rehabilitation centers, nursing homes, sports facilities, and academic institutions.

Patients are typically prescribed physical therapy for a specific purpose by a medical doctor, though the majority of states allow therapists to practice without a physician's referral. Physical therapists treat just about any type of physical dysfunction. In some cases, the problem is the result of illness, such as loss of a leg due to complications of diabetes, or trauma, such as a car accident or sports injury. In other cases, it can be the result of a genetic abnormality, developmental delay, or even simply the effects of aging.

In addition to treating specific physical problems, physical therapists also focus on injury prevention. They:

* provide home care to teach patients and families how to continue rehab
* teach back-care classes to prevent back pain and injury
* show how to modify the performance of tasks to prevent job-related injuries
* condition athletes to prevent injury and improve performance

WHO PERFORMS IT

Physical therapists are licensed in all states, and there are more than 120,000 licensed practitioners in the United States. The minimum requirements are a four-year college degree in physical therapy from an accredited program.

NEED A SPECIALIST?

Physical therapists may become certified in various areas through the American Board of Physical Therapy Specialties. Currently, the board recognizes seven specialities:

* Cardiopulmonary
* Clinical electrophysiology
* Geriatrics
* Neurology
* Orthopedics
* Pediatrics
* Sports physical therapy

POLARITY THERAPY

Polarity therapy is distinguished from other types of energy healing by the broadness of its scope. Though bodywork based on energy theory is the hallmark of polarity therapy, it also incorporates nutrition counseling, an exercise program, and psychological counseling.

HISTORY

Randolph Stone, a chiropractic, osteopathic, and naturopathic physician, created polarity therapy in the mid-1900s. Fascinated by healing modalities of other cultures, he traveled the world to learn their secrets. He studied traditional Chinese medicine, India's Ayurvedic medicine, and ancient Egyptian teachings.

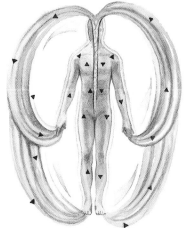

Stone found that underlying the healing practices of all these cultures was a fundamental belief in a universal life force that flowed through every living being. Stagnation or weakness in this energy caused illness, while free-flowing, balanced energy led to good health. The traditional cultures also held that healers did not cure disease; rather, they helped stimulate the body's natural self-healing abilities.

Blending these traditional concepts, Stone developed the theories underlying polarity therapy, which maintains that energy fields exist throughout nature and that free-flowing, balanced energy is fundamental to optimal health. Stone retired in the early 1970s and appointed one of his students, Pierre Pannetier, as his successor. Pannetier led the polarity movement until he died in 1984. The next year, a group of Pannetier's students founded the American Polarity Therapy Association, which created standards of practice and organized practitioner education programs.

WHAT IT IS

According to polarity therapy, energy has a positive, negative, or neutral charge. This does not mean that energy is good or bad, simply that it has one of the three charge states. All of nature is composed of life energy that pulsates back and forth between positive and negative poles, with various neutral areas in between.

In humans, the head is a positive pole, and the feet are a negative pole. The left side of the body is positively charged and the right is negatively charged. In health, energy flows throughout the body in three-dimensional currents. Illness occurs when this flow becomes blocked or imbalanced. The goal of polarity therapy is to balance this flow between positive and negative poles.

Among other modalities, polarity therapists rely primarily on hands-on touch. As with other types of energy healing, the practitioner does not impart his own energy to the patient but instead redirects the flow of the patient's own energy.

The patient remains dressed while lying on a padded table. Using a repertoire of 22 different positions, the practitioner places his hands on various energy centers. The therapist's touch is based on the idea of polarity in that he places his right hand—which is negatively charged—on a positively charged point and

ENERGY CENTERS

According to polarity therapy, energy flows clockwise in the body, passing along a central channel that is neutral. This channel contains five neutral energy centers, each of which is associated with one of five elements: ether, air, fire, water, and earth. These elements are the same as those that are fundamental to traditional Chinese medicine, which maintains that all of nature is composed of these elements. In polarity therapy:

✳ ether regulates the throat and hearing
✳ air controls breathing and the lungs, circulation, and the heart
✳ fire controls digestion
✳ water regulates the glands and emotions
✳ earth controls elimination

his left—or positively charged—hand on a negatively charged point. These positions encourage flow by strengthening healthy energy channels.

The therapist does not manipulate the tissue or bones per se, but instead uses holding, rocking, and vibrating movements that fall into three basic types of touch (based on ancient Ayurvedic concepts):

* *Sattvic touch* is very light. It is used to help the practitioner assess the energy flow and to balance the flow.
* *Rajasic touch* may be gentle or deep and stimulates the body.
* *Tamasic touch* is a pressure that can be quite deep and disperses congested energy.

Stone strongly believed that food has energetic qualities and that proper diet is essential to balancing energy flow. At the beginning of treatment, patients are often counseled to follow a cleansing diet to flush out toxins. The long-term eating pattern polarity therapy encourages is primarily vegetarian.

Polarity yoga is a series of exercises that clients perform on their own. Based on traditional yoga, the exercises involve stretches that enhance the flow of energy.

Because the release of physical tension often leads to emotional release as well, polarity therapy may also involve an element of psychological counseling. Therapists emphasize the power of positive thinking as being essential to creating good health.

USES

Polarity therapy has not been subject to clinical trials. Its benefits are based mainly on anecdotal reports from practitioners and patients. Among the reputed benefits of polarity therapy are:

* relaxation, which alleviates conditions exacerbated by stress
* pain reduction
* heightened self-awareness

WHO PERFORMS IT

There is no licensure for polarity therapists, but the American Polarity Therapy Association (APTA) requires practitioners to meet certain eligibility requirements before obtaining a membership. The APTA has different training requirements for associate practitioners and registered practitioners, who must complete about 300 more hours of study than associates. There are more than 150 APTA members.

REFLEXOLOGY

It may look like a simple foot massage, but reflexology is more than a way to relax. Reflexologists believe that every part of the body is connected to a point in the feet and the hands. Applying pressure to specific points stimulates the body's self-healing abilities, which, in turn, can alleviate a variety of ailments.

HISTORY

The origins of reflexology are as old as those of acupuncture, which dates back well over 2,000 years. Evidence also shows that ancient cultures in Egypt, India, China, and Japan used different forms of foot massage that centered on improving the flow of life energy through various pathways in the body.

Modern-day Western reflexology was initially developed in the early part of this century by American physician William Fitzgerald—an ear, nose, and throat specialist from Connecticut who became interested in what he called *zone theory* while working at a hospital in London. There he learned about the ideas of a British neurologist who had mapped out reflex zones on the head, which were believed to be connected to other areas of the body.

Fitzgerald focused primarily on reflex zones in the hands. He found that by exerting pressure on various points he could avoid using anesthesia during minor surgical procedures. Zone theory gained further popularity when a colleague of Fitzgerald conducted an experiment in which he pressed a spot on a patient's hand, then inserted a needle into the patient's face; the patient felt no pain.

In the 1930s, physical therapist Eunice Ingham took these ideas a step further. While Fitzgerald's zone theory focused on alleviating pain, Ingham believed that the concept had wider applications. Ingham maintained that the feet's sensitivity made them especially responsive to greater therapeutic effects than pain reduction. She developed foot reflexology through years of experimentation on patients, manipulating points on the feet and keeping copious notes of the effects on various parts of the body.

Eventually, Ingham created a detailed map of the feet, connecting points to certain organs, glands, and body parts. She published her first book on her findings in 1938 and went on to create the International Institute of Reflexology, an educational organization that continues to thrive.

WHAT IT IS

The theory behind reflexology is that every part of the body is connected to a pressure point in the ears, hands, and feet. According to reflexology, the entire body is divided into ten zones. These zones run vertically from the top of the head to the toes; there are five zones on the right side and five on the left. By exerting pressure in one area of the zone, a practitioner can alter the energy in another part of the same zone.

Like the body, the sole of each foot is divided into five vertical zones that run from toe to heel, and each of these zones is connected to a zone in the body. Furthermore, the feet are like a miniature version of the body:

- The toes correspond to the head.
- The balls of the feet correspond to the shoulders.
- The arches of the foot correspond to the waist.
- The tops of the heels correspond to the pelvis.
- The bottoms of the heels correspond to the feet.

Any organ, gland, or body part can be found within this map of the feet. For example, the sinuses are found on the big toes, the stomach on the balls of the foot, and the small intestines in the center of the

A HIGH-PROFILE CASE

One of the more famous proponents of reflexology is TV talk show host Regis Philbin. Suffering from a kidney stone that doctors told him was too large to pass, Philbin lay in a New York City hospital bed awaiting surgery. His wife decided to call a leading reflexologist, who came to Philbin's hospital room the night before the operation. She worked on him for about an hour, and within 12 hours he had passed the stone on his own.

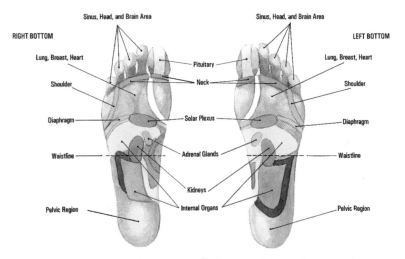

RIGHT BOTTOM

Sinus, Head, and Brain Area

Lung, Breast, Heart

Shoulder

Diaphragm

Waistline

Pelvic Region

Pituitary

Neck

Solar Plexus

Adrenal Glands

Kidneys

Internal Organs

Sinus, Head, and Brain Area

LEFT BOTTOM

Lung, Breast, Heart

Shoulder

Diaphragm

Waistline

Pelvic Region

heels. By working on the appropriate area of the foot, a reflexologist can affect any area of the body.

Also, given their position at the bottom of the body, the feet become a reservoir of toxins. Gravity pushes blood down to the feet, where it tends to stagnate, rather than making its journey back up to the heart. Among these toxins are crystals formed by uric acid, the same chemical found in kidney stones. These toxins interfere with nerve function in the feet, causing congestion in the body part connected to that nerve. Reflexology holds that breaking up these deposits improves circulation, helping the body rid itself of toxins.

Reflexology is more than just a foot massage. The practitioner first strokes and manipulates the feet to relax them and find areas of tenderness. Typically, these areas signal dysfunction in the body parts connected to them, so the practitioner concentrates on these areas, exerting deep pressure with the fingers, thumbs, and palms.

USES

Reflexology improves circulation of blood and lymph, the fluid that carries white blood cells and is important to the immune system. Because points on the feet are connected to every part of the body, reflexologists say it can benefit nearly any condition. The goal, however, is not to cure the ailment but to stimulate the body to heal itself.

The main benefits of reflexology are stress reduction and

relaxation, which in turn benefits just about any health condition made worse by stress, including:

* low-back pain
* gastrointestinal disorders
* headaches
* high blood pressure

Few clinical trials of reflexology have been conducted, but one study that looked at the effect of reflexology on nearly 40 symptoms of premenstrual syndrome (PMS) found that it provided more than twice the level of relief as a placebo treatment. Furthermore, unlike standard hormone and antidepressant medications, reflexology had no side effects.

WHO PERFORMS IT

A variety of health care practitioners use reflexology in their work, including chiropractors, massage therapists, and podiatrists. Because the medical establishment does not view reflexology as a valid treatment, however, there is no licensure specifically for this therapy. The International Institute of Reflexology certifies practitioners who complete formal instruction and pass written and practical tests. More than 25,000 reflexologists are affiliated with the institute.

Reflexology tends to focus on the feet for a variety of reasons. For one thing, the soles of the feet each contain more than 7,000 nerve endings, making them extremely sensitive. The palms of the hands also are rich with nerve endings, but because they are so exposed to use all day, they become desensitized.

REIKI

Besides promoting health and well-being, reiki (pronounced ray-key) aims to help patients reach a higher level of consciousness. Practitioners believe that the therapy causes the body's molecules to vibrate, which dissolves energy blockages that cause illness.

HISTORY

Reiki is a rather mysterious healing technique that is believed to have origins in ancient spiritual practices of Tibetan monks. Modern-day reiki originated in the 1800s with Mikao Usui, a professor of Christian theology in Japan. One day Usui's students asked him a question that thoroughly baffled him. Pointing out that Jesus healed with his hands and instructed his disciples to follow this practice, they challenged him to show them how to heal. This led him on a decades-long quest to learn the secrets of healing.

Usui spent several years at the University of Chicago studying with Christian scholars, but to no avail. Next, he sought out ancient Hindu texts in India, again finding no answers. Finally, he ended up back in Japan, where a Zen Buddhist monk told him that he might find the guidance he was seeking in some ancient Sanskrit Buddhist texts.

After studying the texts, Usui trekked to the top of a holy mountain, where he fasted and meditated for several weeks. Finally, in the dark hours of early morning, he was struck by a dazzling white light, in the midst of which appeared some Sanskrit characters. These characters revealed to Usui the secret of healing, which he called reiki (from the Japanese words *rei*, meaning "free passage," and *ki*, meaning "universal life energy"—like the Chinese *qi*, or *chi*). Shortly after this experience, he performed a series of healing miracles.

Usui traveled throughout Japan, healing and teaching his technique to others, who were called reiki masters. Before he died, Usui appointed his replacement as Grand Master of Reiki, Chujiru Hayashi. Unfortunately, the events of World War II killed all the reiki masters trained by Usui and Hayashi, with the exception of one woman, Hawayo Takata; the therapy survives today solely because of her.

Afflicted with several life-threatening diseases while only in her early 30s, Takata journeyed from her home in Hawaii to die in Japan, birthplace of her ancestors. After she arrived, she received a divine message to go to Hayashi's clinic, where reiki treatment cured her. She was initiated as a reiki master in the late 1930s, then returned to Hawaii to practice. After Hayashi died, she became Grand Master, eventually training 21 other masters. These masters in turn trained other masters, and today there are about 1,000 masters around the world.

WHAT IT IS

Reiki is a universal, high-vibration energy that animates all levels of existence: physical, mental, emotional, and spiritual. Reiki has an intelligence of its own, and its action is always positive.

In most people, the flow of reiki energy becomes blocked over time, which can cause physical and emotional dysfunction. Although everyone has the potential to tap into reiki, one must be trained in this ability. Thus, in most cases, a reiki practitioner must first attune himself to the person's energy field. In order to tap into reiki energy, one must have a master open the person's channels and be trained to accept the frequency of one's own reiki energy field. Once the master has opened the channel for the reiki to flow freely, the individual will be able to tap into the energy himself for the rest of his life.

Reiki practitioners believe that the *chakras*—the Ayurvedic energy centers in the body—are fundamental to reiki's healing power, though no one truly knows why reiki works. Reiki theorists point out that the locations of the various chakras are closely related to the locations of various endocrine glands, which secrete hormones that control metabolism, reproduction, development, and many other essential processes. Reiki practitioners postulate that this close relationship underlies the therapy's ability to heal.

A reiki session usually lasts about an hour. The patient

BECOMING A MASTER

Initiation into reiki is divided into three levels. In the first level, a reiki master guides practitioners to become attuned to reiki energy and learn how to channel it both for themselves and for other people. First-level practitioners then are allowed to perform hands-on healing.

At the second level, the practitioner learns more symbols and furthers his ability to perform hands-on treatment. The practitioner also learns how to perform absentee treatment, which involves attuning oneself to reiki energy in a subject who is not present, for instance, by using a photograph of the person.

Third-degree practitioners learn a final symbol that enables them to become reiki masters. At this level, a master is able to initiate others into the therapy and also experiences increased power of his own treatments.

remains fully clothed while lying on his back on a flat surface. Beginning at the top of the head and moving downward, the practitioner very gently places her hands on the patient's body, leaving them in position for about five minutes before moving them to a new area; she keeps her hands still. Practitioners use about 20 hand positions during a treatment, allowing their intuition to guide them to areas of the body that need unblocking. Patients often report a warm feeling or a sensation of tingling during the treatment.

USES

Reiki has not been the subject of controlled trials. Practition-ers say it can be used for any physical or mental disorder, especially pain and problems related to stress. Patients often say that it leaves them with a heightened sense of self-aware-ness and well-being, and that it causes profound emotional release.

WHO PERFORMS IT

Although individuals are en-couraged to practice reiki on themselves, the therapy cannot be learned from a book. Train-ing in reiki occurs through an intensive initiation process by which participants learn how to use the ancient sounds and symbols revealed to Usui to attune themselves to reiki energy.

ROLFING

Like the Leaning Tower of Pisa, a body that is structurally out of balance will be pulled constantly toward the ground by gravity. There's no escaping this universal force, but Rolfing can help overcome gravity's effects on the body—visible to most of us as sagging and slouching. This intense type of massage has been so influential in the field that it is one of the few types of bodywork to be defined in the dictionary.

HISTORY

Rolfing was developed by Ida Rolf, who received a Ph.D. in biological chemistry from Columbia University's College of Physicians and Surgeons in 1920. Rolf was interested in a variety of unorthodox therapies, including yoga, chiropractic, and osteopathy. During the course of her research and informal studies, Rolf discovered the importance of fascia, the flexible connective tissue that envelops all the muscles and organs in the body. Fascia is what gives the body shape, because it holds everything in place.

Over a person's life, fascia typically becomes distorted from such things as physical injury, poor posture, and even emotional trauma. Fascia adapts to these insults by shortening and thickening, pulling bones, muscles, and organs out of position.

As imbalance occurs in one area of the body, it creates imbalance in others as well. A young child who falls on the playground and injures her leg, for example, may limp for a couple of weeks. Shifting her weight to the other leg affects muscles in the pelvis, spine, and upper body. Even after the limp disappears, a legacy of distorted fascia throughout her body is left behind. Weighted down by gravity, these distortions become more pronounced and problematic over time.

To release these ingrained patterns of tension and imbalance, Rolf, who herself suffered from scoliosis and spinal arthritis, developed a form of deep-tissue massage that she called Structural Integration. (In

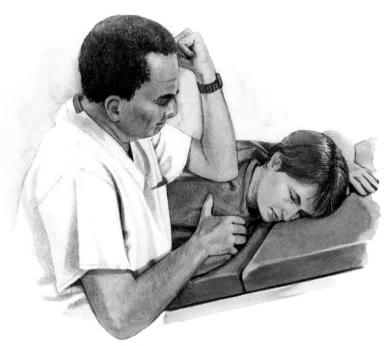

tribute, however, her students preferred to call the technique simply "Rolfing," the name that has stuck.) Rolfing remained fairly obscure until the 1960s, when Rolf began teaching her technique at the Esalen Institute in Big Sur, California, which was the focal point of the burgeoning human potential movement. In 1971—still going strong at age 75—Rolf established the Rolf Institute of Structural Integration in Boulder, Colorado.

WHAT IT IS

Rolfing is aimed at restoring the flexibility and length of the connective tissue, thus alleviat-

ing misalignment in the body. The hallmark of Rolfing is what is called the *Rolf line*. In a properly aligned body, a straight line drawn from a person's head to feet should intersect with the midpoint of the ears, shoulder joints, hip joints, knees, and ankles. In a typical patient, however, a line drawn through these midpoints is curvy, indicating misalignment.

The basic Rolfing series consists of ten sessions of approximately one hour, with each session building on the work of the last one. For most of the work, the patient lies on a padded table. To increase friction, the Rolfer does not use oil as he uses his fingers, hands, fists, and elbows to manipulate the fascia and release adhesions. The goal is not for the practitioner to move the fascia, but to release tension and then help the client develop more efficient movement patterns that work with, rather than against, gravity. Rolfers often give patients exercises to perform at home.

Before the series begins, the patient is photographed in his underwear to help evaluate distortions in the Rolf line. The first session focuses on releasing restriction in the shoulders, chest, lower back, and pelvis, which helps improve circulation and respiration. The second session concentrates on freeing restrictions from the feet to the knees, leading to more even weight distribution. The third session removes tension from the sides of the body and begins to work toward improving the Rolf line at the body's core.

Session four begins the deep-tissue work for which Rolfing is renowned. The remaining sessions continue this work, concentrating on the following areas:

- improving weight transmission through the inner legs and up the pelvis and spine
- releasing fascial restrictions on internal organs
- liberating muscles along the spine
- improving the relationship between the head and neck and the rest of the body
- bringing the body into balance from side to side, front to back, and inside to out
- polishing the balancing and integrative process

After completion of the series, the patient is photographed again and the practitioner assesses the Rolf line one more time.

USES

Clinical studies of Rolfing have been limited, but research has found that it:

- reduces stress and anxiety
- strengthens the body's physical structure
- improves posture
- improves nervous system functioning

Practitioners also say it eases low-back pain and enhances everyday physical performance. Comparison of before and after pictures of the Rolf line can reveal significant differences, including improved alignment

ROLFING THE STARS

Many famous people have undergone Rolfing, including Cary Grant, Georgia O'Keeffe, and Greta Garbo. Garbo was treated by Ida Rolf herself, but Garbo initially wasn't pleased with the results. Convinced that Rolf had changed the shape of her face and made her mouth bigger, she threatened to sue. Garbo was placated, however, when Cecil Beaton, photographer to the stars, photographed her and told her that her looks actually had improved.

and posture, decreased sagging of skin and muscles, and a more relaxed appearance. Many patients report that people tell them they look years younger and several inches taller.

Because Rolfing is a therapy that treats the whole person, patients often find it relieves not just long-standing physical aches and pains but emotional pain as well.

WHO PERFORMS IT

Though Ida Rolf feared that no one would continue her practice after she died, which she did in 1979, today there are around 850 Rolfers around the world. To use the title "Rolfer," a practitioner must be trained and certified by the Rolf Institute. To be accepted into the program, students must have an extensive background in anatomy, physiology, and kinesiology, as well as some background in psychology, which helps them deal with emotional issues that may arise for patients during the sessions. The Rolf program involves hundreds of hours of course work, observation, and hands-on practice.

There are a number of Rolfing "spin-offs." Most were started by people trained in Rolfing but developed ideas and techniques that do not conform with Rolfing orthodoxy.

SHIATSU

Closely related to acupressure, shiatsu is a fairly recent development, given that it is based on the principles of traditional Chinese medicine, which date back several thousand years. Shiatsu, however, was created only in the early part of the 1900s.

HISTORY

Tradition has it that about 1,000 years ago, a Buddhist priest introduced Chinese medicine to Japan. Out of traditional Chinese concepts grew a Japanese form of massage called amma, which involved pressing and rubbing techniques. Amma was primarily performed by the blind, because they were generally believed to have a heightened sense of touch.

In the early part of the 20th century, high-tech Western medicine began to exert an increasing level of influence on the Japanese aristocracy, and the government cracked down on the practice of amma. New licensing laws attempted to limit traditional medicine and also control illicit massage practices. In response to the governmental controls, legitimate amma practitioners began calling their practice shiatsu— meaning "finger pressure"—in order to avoid licensing regulations.

But shiatsu too was almost eliminated. After World War II, General Douglas MacArthur branded shiatsu as unscientific and banned it along with other traditional healing methods. Because shiatsu was still a traditional source of livelihood for the blind, the Japanese Blind Association appealed to Helen Keller for help. Keller persuaded President Truman to reverse the ban, and shiatsu was free to flourish.

One of the most important shiatsu practitioners was Tokujiro Namikoshi, who owned a shiatsu school in Tokyo. Namikoshi helped set shiatsu apart from amma as its own modality by bringing in sighted practitioners, describing it in Western terms, and simplifying the techniques. Like acupressure, shiatsu was introduced to

The Healing Power of Touch

the West after journalist James Reston's experience with acupuncture for pain related to an emergency appendectomy he had in China in the early 1970s.

WHAT IT IS

As in Chinese medicine, Japanese medicine recognizes a life energy—called *ki* in Japanese rather than the Chinese *qi*—that flows through all living beings. Ki flows throughout the entire body along 12 main channels, called meridians, each associated with a particular organ. As it flows throughout the body, ki may become excessive or weak in certain areas. Practitioners can build up weak ki or release excess ki by stimulating hundreds of points called *tsubos*, which are located along the meridians.

The practitioner generally uses her knuckles, palms, elbows, or even feet to apply pressure to the points, and the pressure may be light or deep, depending on the desired affect. Shiatsu pressure is generally applied for three to five seconds.

Shiatsu practitioners use a couple of different techniques. Some focus on certain *tsubos*, while others take a more general approach, using pressure all over the body to stimulate balanced flow of ki throughout the meridians.

USES

There isn't much scientific research specifically on shiatsu, but it is believed that findings on acupressure, acupuncture, and massage are relevant to this therapy as well. Practitioners believe that shiatsu is effective as a general tonic to enhance

WHAT'S THE DIFFERENCE?

Acupressure and shiatsu are so closely related that some sources make no distinction between the two. However, there are a couple of key differences:

❋ Though both therapies involve pressure on points that fall along energy meridians in the body, acupressure is applied only to the points of acupuncture, of which there are about 360. Shiatsu is used on 660 points.

❋ Acupressure is lighter and longer; points may be held for as long as three minutes. Shiatsu pressure is firmer and more vigorous, and is applied for only three to five seconds.

health and as a treatment that stimulates the body's ability to heal itself in cases of specific illness.

Although shiatsu can be very helpful in alleviating some of the discomforts of pregnancy, especially morning sickness, pregnant women should not use shiatsu without the advice of a health care practitioner. Pressure on certain points has shown to cause uterine contractions and may lead to miscarriage.

Shiatsu should also be avoided if you have a heart condition, after a heavy meal or exertion, in cases of acute infection, or on points where there is a bruise, open wound, mole, wart, or varicose vein.

WHO PERFORMS IT

Many massage schools train practitioners in shiatsu. Additionally, the American Oriental Bodywork Therapy Association certifies practitioners in oriental bodywork, which includes shiatsu.

Sports Massage

Besides Michael Jordan, what gives the Chicago Bulls basketball team their winning edge? It could be their use of sports massage. The team's strength coach has said it's one of the most important things the organization has done for the team, because it helps prevent injury and speed recovery.

HISTORY

Massage has long been used in Eastern Europe to boost athletic performance. Sports massage initially came to the United States by way of a French military base during World War II. Jack Meagher, a physical therapist stationed there as a soldier, became interested in the technique after a German prisoner of war gave him pregame massages to enhance his performance during football games on the base. After the war, Meagher played professional baseball but was forced out of the sport by an old injury to his shoulder. Massage to the area improved his baseball performance to the point where he could play again as a semipro. Meagher developed a reputation for using massage therapy to treat various sports injuries. In the early 1980s, he began to pass on his techniques to younger massage therapists who were part of the resurgence of massage.

Sports massage didn't receive recognition in this country, however, until several decades later, when it was offered to athletes at the 1984 Olympic Games in Los Angeles. In 1985, the American Massage Therapy Association (AMTA) established its National Sports Massage Certification Program and created the AMTA National Sports Massage Team. This team comprises more than 300 practitioners who travel with various professional and collegiate sports teams and have provided their services at major events, such as the Goodwill Games, the Boston Marathon, and the Ironman Triathalon. In 1996, sports massage was included for the first time as part of the medical services provided at the Olympic Games in Atlanta and was available at all event venues.

WHAT IT IS

The primary goals of sports massage are to prevent injury, maximize performance, and aid in the recovery from injury. Although practitioners of sports massage do use strokes from Swedish massage, they rely primarily on two additional techniques: compression and direct pressure.

In compression, the therapist uses his fingers, palm, or fist to spread the muscle against the underlying bone. This increases circulation and prepares the athlete for optimal performance. Compression is used only on bony areas, such as the arms and legs.

With direct pressure, the therapist uses his fingers and thumbs to apply pressure repeatedly on a tight or painful area. This, too, helps stimulate circulation and soften the muscle tissue. Direct pressure may also involve friction, in which the therapist strokes a muscle perpendicularly to the direction in which the muscle runs. Friction helps break down adhesions and reduce spasms, increasing flexibility.

Hydrotherapy and ice therapy are commonly used as adjunct treatments to sports massage. Hydrotherapy is any therapy involving water, such as whirlpools and steam rooms. Applying ice to an area can reduce swelling and pain.

USES

The focus of a sports massage session depends on when it is being performed. A maintenance program of massage aims to keep an athlete injury free and performing at peak level. A sports massage therapist knows which muscles are likely to cause trouble in a given sport and focuses on those muscles, improving their flexibility and range of motion.

Sports massage is often administered immediately before and up to two hours after an athletic event. Prior to performance, the massage is meant to enhance warm-up by increasing circulation and reducing muscle tension. After an event, the goal is to reduce muscle spasms and ease stiffness by removing lactic acid from the tissues. (Lactic acid is a waste product created by vigorous exercise; it is one of the major causes of cramping.) During training, sports massage can reduce soreness and enable an athlete to train more.

Despite the best preventive efforts, injuries are simply a fact of nearly any athletic endeavor.

The Healing Power of Touch

DEEP-TISSUE MASSAGE

Although you may have heard of deep-tissue massage as a particular school of massage therapy, it's really a more general term for a technique incorporated in many kinds of practice. In contrast to Swedish massage, which focuses on superficial layers of muscle, deep-tissue work concentrates on manipulating lower, or deeper, layers. It can be particularly useful in treating a dysfunction or chronic tension in an isolated part of the body, such as neck or ankle pain. A therapist must be highly skilled and knowledgeable to be effective at deep-tissue massage.

Sports massage can reduce pain and speed healing during rehabilitation. Direct pressure techniques, for instance, alleviate spasms, while friction can help reduce the formation of scar tissue. Specific injuries helped by massage include:

* *Sprains:* Massage above and below the sprain aids removal of waste products to reduce swelling. After several days, massage is used to stimulate circulation and aid proper movement.
* *Muscle Tears/Strains:* In cases of small tears, massage can improve circulation in the damaged area and help recovery and reduce scar tissue.
* *Bruising:* Bruises occur when blood vessels rupture and there is nowhere for blood to go. Massage improves circulation around the bruise.

WHO PERFORMS IT

The American Massage Therapy Association (AMTA) administers written and practical exams to certify practitioners in sports massage. The AMTA's National Sports Massage Team is made up of more than 300 certified practitioners who are qualified to work at pre- and postcompetition stages of athletic events.

SWEDISH MASSAGE

When most people think of massage, they think of the classic Swedish massage, which is perhaps the most popular form of bodywork in the world. A deeply relaxing therapy, Swedish massage is the foundation for many techniques of contemporary Western massage. And it does more than calm the mind: Research shows it alleviates pain, eases nausea, boosts immunity, and increases weight gain in premature infants.

HISTORY

Massage may very well be the oldest form of health care in the world. Egyptian tomb paintings depict people receiving massage, ancient Chinese and Indian texts refer to it as a treatment for disease and injury, and Greek and Roman physicians relied on it as one of their primary therapies.

Swedish massage was developed in the early 1800s by Swedish fencing master and gymnastics instructor Per Henrik Ling. Ling sought to create a type of body manipulation that echoed the benefits of Swedish gymnastics, an exercise regimen also developed by Ling consisting of 800 movements that increased circulation and muscle tone and balanced the body.

Ling based his technique on scientific knowledge of anatomy and physiology. Like many other healers throughout history, Ling's interest in massage was due in part to having a health problem himself: The bodywork he created—which he called the Swedish Movement Cure—relieved his rheumatism.

The Swedish government was less than enthusiastic about Ling's therapy, however. When, in 1812, he applied for a license to teach his technique, the government rejected his request. Nevertheless, popular demand for Ling's treatment was so great that two years later his application was granted and his school was supported by a grant from the King of Sweden.

Swedish massage eventually spread to other parts of the Western world, and today it serves as the basis for many other types of bodywork, including sports massage, trigger-point therapy, and infant massage.

WHAT IT IS

Patients remove as much clothing as feels comfortable to them. They remain covered with a sheet or towel, except for the part of the body the therapist is working on. Breasts and genitals are not massaged.

Swedish massage tends to concentrate on superficial muscle layers, rather than deep-tissue work; the goal is to stimulate circulation of blood and movement of the lymph. Five basic strokes form the foundation of Swedish massage. Practitioners of Swedish massage generally combine these five techniques and work on the entire body, using oil to help their hands glide more easily over the skin.

✳ Effleurage, which means "touching lightly," is a smooth, gliding stroke that the practitioner generally uses to begin and end the session. This stroke, which can be superficial or deep, allows the therapist to assess the patient's soft tissues, that is, muscles, ligaments, tendons, and connective tissue. It also warms and relaxes the tissue, preparing it for the massage session. It is done in the direction of the heart, to stimulate circulation of blood and movement of the lymph, the fluid that carries white blood cells and is important to the immune system. Increasing circulation helps remove waste products and reduce inflammation.

✳ Petrissage, or "kneading," lifts muscles away from bone, then rolls and kneads them, like bread dough. Petrissage also stimulates circulation of blood and lymph.

✳ Friction ("rubbing"), the deepest of the five strokes, involves deep circular or transverse strokes that cause layers of tissue to rub against one another. The goal of friction is to break down adhesions and make muscles and joints more supple. Friction also increases blood flow to a specific area where it is applied.

✳ Tapotement ("tapping") is also known as percussion or pounding. Typically using the edge of her hands, the therapist strikes the patient's body with rapid, alternating blows. The affects of percussion vary according to the length of time the stroke is applied. When administered for less than 10 seconds, it is stimulating; when applied for a longer period, of up to a minute, it is relaxing. More than 60 seconds of tapotment fatigues the muscles, which can be beneficial for those that are cramped or in spasm.

* The last type of stroke is vibration ("shaking"), which, like tapotement, can be either stimulating or relaxing, depending on how long it is performed. The practitioner uses shaking movements with her hand or fingers, which are especially useful for stimulating the nerves.

USES

Modern-day research proves that the ancients knew what they were doing: Among many other findings, studies show that massage eases stress and depression, alleviates muscle and joint disorders, and reduces pain. Massage has been shown to induce the relaxation response, a profoundly relaxed state in which heart rate and blood pressure decrease and brain waves slow down. Massage also causes the release of endorphins, neurochemicals that alleviate pain and produce a sense of well-being.

The therapeutic effects of massage are vast indeed. Among its many scientifically documented benefits, massage:

* improves the movement of lymph, the fluid that removes

water and carries white blood cells and is important to immunity
* decreases muscle pain and tension
* alleviates tension headaches and post-traumatic headaches
* reduces traumatically induced spinal pain
* alleviates carpal tunnel syndrome
* eases symptoms of fibromyalgia, a condition of chronic muscular pain
* decreases pain and disability in patients with inflammatory bowel disease
* promotes relaxation and comfort in hospice patients
* alleviates pain and anxiety in cancer patients
* reduces nausea from chemotherapy
* increases immune function in HIV patients
* increases weight gain in premature infants
* increases the time premature infants are awake and active
* decreases depression and anxiety in children and teenagers
* decreases types of autistic behavior in children with autism
* reduces nausea in pregnant women

* alleviates breast tenderness and engorgement after giving birth
* decreases the need for episiotomy in childbirth
* improves self-image and decreases depression in women with bulimia

WHO PERFORMS IT

Currently, it is estimated that there are as many as 150,000 massage therapists in the United States. Massage therapists are licensed in 25 states and the District of Columbia. In the remaining states, local government bodies generally regulate the practice. In addition, the National Certification Board for Therapeutic Massage and Bodywork certifies practitioners.

Because licensing is not available to all practitioners, you may want to ask whether a therapist is affiliated with an organization such as the American Massage Therapy Association (AMTA), which has stringent guidelines for membership, including, at a minimum, completion of an accredited massage therapy program. AMTA has more than 30,000 members in more than 24 countries.

THERAPEUTIC TOUCH

Though the medical establishment is still skeptical of Therapeutic Touch's benefits, it has become extremely popular among nurses in the United States, who use it to ease anxiety and even treat pain in their patients.

HISTORY

Therapeutic Touch has much in common with the ancient practice known as laying on of hands. Fifteen-thousand-year-old cave paintings in the Pyrenees mountains show humans healing by laying their hands on others, and the practice was common in early Christian times. St. Patrick, for instance, healed the blind with his hands.

In the 1970s, a retired Hungarian military colonel named Oskar Estebany became world renowned for his power to heal both people and animals with his hands. This ability of Estebany, who was known simply as Mr. E, first came to light when he was in the cavalry and his horse fell ill. He spent the night massaging it; the next day, the horse was cured.

Mr. E's method was subjected to study by scientists at McGill University, who found that he decreased the healing time for wounded mice. Two nurses, Dolores Krieger, Ph.D., professor emerita of nursing at New York University, and Dora Kunz, a clairvoyant and healer, spent a great deal of time observing Mr. E and were amazed by his results. He simply sat quietly with patients, gently laying his hands on the places that he felt needed healing. Based on their studies of Mr. E and other healers, Krieger and Kunz founded the modality known as Therapeutic Touch.

WHAT IT IS

According to Therapeutic Touch, human beings are composed not simply of matter but also of electromagnetic energy, which permeates and surrounds the body in an invisible field. Energy from the environment enters this field of energy, circulates through the system, then leaves.

This idea is similar to ancient Hindu teachings, which hold that the human body contains

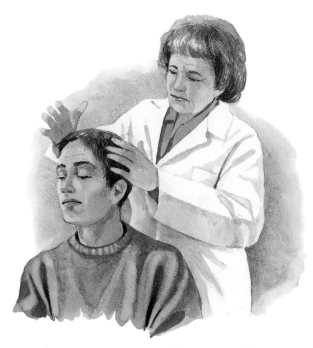

seven energy centers, called *chakras*. Chakras take in vital life energy, or *prana*, and enable the body to use it. *Prana* circulates through the *chakras* and eventually leaves the body.

Each person's pattern and amount of energy is unique, though everyone has in common the fact that their right and left sides are mirror images of one another. In a person who is ill, the symmetry of the energy configuration is thrown off and the person's overall energy is depleted, whereas a healthy person has a balanced pattern of energy and an excess amount of it.

Therapeutic Touch practitioners do not diagnose specific conditions; instead, they use their intuition to sense areas of low or blocked energy, then focus on building up and smoothing the energy flow. The Therapeutic Touch practitioner helps reorganize the pattern of energy in the patient, working toward a configuration that is balanced and whole.

During a Therapeutic Touch session, which usually lasts about a half hour, the patient remains fully clothed while sitting in a chair, so the practitioner can easily access all sides of the body. The session is then conducted in the following stages.

* *Centering:* At the beginning of the session, the practitioner engages in a few moments of quiet meditation or deep breathing. This establishes the intent and compassion to heal. Centering also helps the practitioner connect with her own source of energy and become focused, which, in turn, enables her to attune herself to the energy field of the patient, more correctly called the receiver.

* *Assessment:* The therapist stands and then kneels in front of the receiver as she rapidly passes her hands several inches away from the body, palms facing the receiver. Then she repeats this in back of the receiver. A healthy person's field will feel whole and unbroken. In an unhealthy person, the practitioner may feel hot or cold spots, a tingling feeling, or even just an intuitive sense that there is an imbalance.

* *Unruffling:* The goal is to release blocked energy and enable it to flow freely. The practitioner repeatedly moves her hands down the receiver's body in rhythmic, sweeping motions, again holding her hands several inches away from the body. At the end of each stroke, she shakes the energy off her fingers, like shaking off water.

* *Transferring energy:* Here the practitioner aims to fill in areas where she sensed a deficit of energy. Despite the name of this stage, the practitioner does not give away her own energy. Rather, she is a conduit for universal energy and simply directs this energy to the receiver. She positions her hands near weak spots, directing energy to flow there.

USES

Although critics point out that the very existence of bio-energy fields isn't conclusively proven, let alone the effects of using these fields in medical treatment, a number of studies have documented positive effects from Therapeutic Touch. Of all the types of biofield therapeutics, this is the best studied.

Therapeutic Touch has been found to induce the relaxation response—a deeply relaxed state in which heart rate and blood pressure decline and brain waves slow down. The relaxation response can benefit any health condition exacerbated by stress.

The Healing Power of Touch

MORE ENERGY HEALING

A couple of other biofield therapies also are practiced in the United States.

❊ *Healing Touch:* Also developed by a nurse, this therapy uses Therapeutic Touch as a foundation but also incorporates other techniques, including *chakra* connection and magnetic unruffling. The therapy has been incorporated by the American Holistic Nurses' Association, which offers a four-level certification program.

❊ *SHEN:* An acronym for Specific Human Energy Nexus, SHEN aims to release painful emotions that are embedded in the body and cause physical effects. Without exerting pressure, the practitioner uses a series of paired-hand positions to discover the location of embedded emotions in the patient. Energy flows from the practitioner's hands through the emotional centers of the patient's body to discharge the emotions, which flow out of the body and are replaced by feelings of love, joy, and confidence.

Among the conditions that have been studied are:

❊ *Wound Healing:* One study looked at identical surgically induced minor wounds in young men. The group that received Therapeutic Touch healed significantly faster than the group that did not.

❊ *Anxiety:* Studies of Therapeutic Touch performed on cardiac patients have found that it reduces anxiety and blood pressure.

❊ *Pain:* Research has found that Therapeutic Touch reduces tension headaches, premenstrual syndrome, and post-surgical pain.

Additionally, Therapeutic Touch is increasingly being used with terminally ill and dying patients.

WHO PERFORMS IT

Therapeutic Touch is widely taught to health care professionals, mainly nurses. In fact, discussion of the therapy is included in most basic nursing textbooks. It is estimated that as many as 30,000 health care professionals practice Therapeutic Touch around the world. Laypeople can also learn Therapeutic Touch for home use.

TRAGER APPROACH

What sets the Trager Approach apart from other forms of movement re-education is its emphasis on mind-to-muscle communication from practitioner to patient. Though they use hands-on touch, Trager therapists place equal emphasis on their own state of mind during treatment, which helps effect change in patients.

HISTORY

As a teenage boxer in the 1920s, Milton Trager discovered his healing abilities purely by accident. One day, Trager's trainer, who gave him daily rubdowns, traded places with him. The trainer told Trager that he had a real flair for hands-on healing, which was confirmed when Trager went home and attempted to try treating his father's sciatica. When the pain disappeared after only a couple of days, Trager decided to pursue a career as a healer.

For nearly a decade he developed his approach by working with patients who had debilitating illnesses, such as polio. Trager went on to work in the physical therapy department of the U.S. Navy during World War II, and when the war was over he decided to become a doctor. However, all the U.S. medical schools he applied to rejected him, contending that at age 42, he was too old to enter the profession. He finally earned his medical degree in Mexico and moved to Hawaii, where he quietly practiced for nearly two decades. His work won notoriety after he was invited to teach at the Esalen Institute in Big Sur, California.

Eventually, in 1980, Trager cofounded the Trager Institute in Mill Valley, California, which teaches and certifies Trager practitioners.

WHAT IT IS

According to the Trager Approach, the brain is the source of physical dysfunction. Physical or emotional trauma causes the mind to hold muscles in tight, painful positions that block the natural flow of movement in the body. By using hands-on techniques and unspoken communication, the

The Healing Power of Touch

practitioner works in a meditative state called *hook-up*, and it is this state that leads to results.

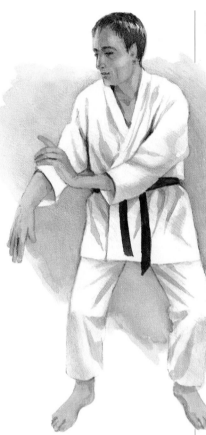

The practitioner uses very light touch to move rhythmically the patient's head, torso, and limbs with gentle rocking and shaking movements—as many as 6,000 movements in an hour-long session. The idea is to give the client the experience of being able to move each part freely and without effort.

After the bodywork, the patient is instructed in what is called *Mentastics*—Trager's word for mental gymnastics. These are a series of simple, dancelike sequences that are aimed at helping clients recreate the sensations experienced during the bodywork. The client is meant to use these exercises at home.

practitioner shows the patient's unconscious mind what lighter, freer movement feels like. The unconscious then becomes the agent of change; remembering and repeating the lessons it learned at the hands of the practitioner, it releases constricted muscle patterns.

Clients lie on a padded table wearing swimwear or underwear, and lubrication is not used. A unique aspect of the Trager Approach is that the

USES

The Trager Approach has not been the subject of much scientific study, so reports on its effectiveness tend to be anecdotal. Patients say that the Trager Approach leaves them with feelings of deep relaxation,

GETTING HOOKED

Though touch is essential to the Trager Approach, practitioners do not try to manipulate or change the tissues of the body. Instead, they focus on communicating a feeling of lightness and freedom to the nervous system. The client's body absorbs the message and that is how change occurs.

Trager therapists communicate this feeling by entering a meditative state that Milton Trager termed *hook-up*. In hook-up, the goal is for the therapist to become one with the energy force that surrounds all life. While in this state, she is able to communicate with the patient's unconscious and convey new patterns of movement.

As she gently rocks and shakes various parts of the client's body, the practitioner's hands silently repeat the questions: "What could be softer? Lighter? Freer?"

The practitioner must eliminate her own thoughts and goals and simply act as a conduit of learning for the patient. Trager theory holds that self-awareness is shaped by sensory experience; when the practitioner inputs positive sensory experience, it naturally replaces the negative sensory experience that led to physical discomfort. This alteration in sensory experience is what creates lasting physical change.

improved physical movement, and greater energy and mental awareness. It is typically used by patients with musculoskeletal problems, which can be caused by multiple sclerosis, cerebral palsy, and stroke or spinal cord injuries. Practitioners have treated thousands of patients with back problems, which tend to respond quite positively to the therapy. Some athletes use it to enhance their performance.

WHO PERFORMS IT

The Trager Institute trains and certifies practitioners who complete its program. In addition to classes on theory and practice of the Trager Approach, anatomy, and physiology, the certification program includes hands-on work and private tutorials. There are approximately 1,000 Trager practitioners around the world.

TRIGGER POINT

If they're not loosened up, tight muscles can give rise to tender, chronically painful areas called trigger points. Not only are these areas themselves hypersensitive, but they can also refer pain to other areas of the body. A trigger point in the shoulder, for instance, may cause headache pain.

HISTORY

Trigger point therapy was pioneered by Janet Travell, M.D., in the late 1930s and early 1940s. As with many other forms of touch therapy, trigger point techniques arose from Travell's personal experience. As she used self-massage on a sore shoulder, she felt pain radiating into her arm. She became interested in this phenomenon of referred pain and, observing patients in her medical practice, discovered that severe muscle pain often was reproduced in other areas of the body, in many cases quite a distance from the original pain.

Through trial and error, Travell was able to map out specific trigger points and referral areas. She also developed a method for treating trigger point pain, called the "spray and stretch" technique (see next page). She won wide acclaim for successfully treating John F. Kennedy's excruciating back pain. Debilitated by war injuries, U.S. senator Kennedy was forced to use crutches because his back pain was so

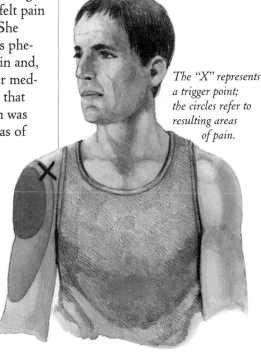

The "X" represents a trigger point; the circles refer to resulting areas of pain.

OTHER TYPES OF TRIGGERS

Janet Travell's "spray and stretch" technique isn't the only type of trigger point therapy. Another well-known system is Bonnie Prudden Myotherapy, a method that desensitizes trigger points with finger, knuckle, or elbow pressure instead of injection with anesthetic. In myotherapy, the patient is asked to rate the degree of pain as pressure is applied, on a scale of one to 10. The practitioner aims to work in the range of six to eight; anything higher will only cause further muscle spasm and be counterproductive. Practitioners can become certified in this technique after taking coursework through the Bonnie Prudden School for Fitness and Myotherapy in Tuscon, Arizona.

bad; surgery afforded him no relief. His transformation to the vigorous, outdoors-loving president everyone remembers occurred thanks to Travell's treatment, which included ergonomic changes in all of his chairs and seats. Her efforts were rewarded when she was named the first female White House physician, serving under Presidents Kennedy and Johnson.

WHAT IT IS

Trigger points are hypersensitive areas that can occur not only in muscles but also in tendons and fascia, the connective tissue that binds muscles and bones and covers all the organs of the body. Applying pressure to these points causes pain in other areas of the body, areas that often are distant from the trigger point.

Trigger points can be caused by a variety of things, including injury, overuse, structural imbalances, and poor posture. As a result of any of these factors, muscles contract. If the contraction becomes chronic, it can cause trigger points, which can reduce strength, flexibility, and range of motion. The goal of trigger point therapy is to release these contractions and eliminate the referred pain.

Travell developed a method called spray and stretch. The practitioner sprays or injects trigger points with anesthesia to desensitize and relax them. This allows the therapist to stretch and massage the area, which improves the circulation of blood and lymph and prevents the trigger point from recurring.

Other methods of trigger point therapy developed out of Travell's technique when it was discovered that finger pressure also could sedate and relax trigger points (see "Other Types of Triggers").

USES

Although clinical study of trigger point therapy is limited, it is a standard part of the curriculum at many massage schools. Neuromuscular massage therapy also includes treatment of trigger points. Practitioners have found trigger point therapy to be especially beneficial in cases of musculoskeletal problems, such as whiplash, tendinitis, bursitis, and temporomandibular disorder (TMD). It may be useful for pain that seems to have no apparent cause but may in fact be radiating from a trigger point, for instance, headaches.

WHO PERFORMS IT

Trigger point therapy is used by massage therapists, chiropractors, physical therapists, and even some conventional medical doctors.

TUI-NA

Tui-na (pronounced tway na) is an ancient Chinese form of acupressure massage. Tui means "to push," and *na* means "to grasp." Based on the principles of traditional Chinese medicine, tui-na aims to balance the flow of *qi*, the vital life force that courses through all of nature.

HISTORY

Reference to tui-na as an important healing modality can be found in *The Yellow Emperor's Classic of Internal Medicine*, a comprehensive text of traditional Chinese medicine that records practices believed to date back more than 4,000 years. By around A.D. 600, tui-na was part of the curriculum of the Imperial College of Medicine. Eventually, the explorer Marco Polo brought tui-na to Europe, and some experts believe this type of bodywork formed the basis of Swedish massage, which was developed in the early 1800s, though there is no evidence to validate this theory. In China, tui-na is a standard part of the program at traditional medical colleges; it is considered as important a modality as acupuncture and herbal medicine. In China today, the term *tui-na* is used to refer to massage therapy generally.

Tui-na was first taught in the United States at the Taoist Institute in Los Angeles in the mid-1970s. As the interest in Chinese medicine, particularly acupuncture, continues to grow in this country, access to tui-na is becoming more readily available, and it has become part of the curriculum at a number of massage schools.

WHAT IT IS

In Chinese medicine, qi is the life energy that flows through all living beings. Qi flows throughout the entire body along 12 main channels, called meridians, each associated with a particular organ. Disease is the result of either excessive or weak qi. Practitioners can build up weak qi or release excess qi by stimulating the hundreds of acupressure points located along the meridians and smaller channels called collaterals.

In tui-na different techniques are used to either sedate (relax) or tonify (stimulate) a particular area, depending on whether the energy there is excessive or deficient. Tui-na was handed down through various medical traditions, and today there are five major approaches to tui-na.

* *The one-finger school* focuses on stimulating acupressure points with the thumb and is used for internal and gynecologic conditions.
* *The rolling school* is based on the one-finger technique but is used on wider parts of the body; it treats soft tissue problems.
* *Flat pushing* is used to channel qi to the patient.
* *Pointing massage* is a form of first-aid medicine based on acupressure.
* *Bonesetting* treats orthopedic problems.

USES

Tui-na is used to treat a wide variety of ailments, including:

* headaches
* insomnia
* asthma
* hayfever
* menstrual cramps
* arthritis
* back pain
* sore throat

WHO PERFORMS IT

Some massage therapists may be trained in tui-na during massage therapy school. Acupuncturists, if they receive a thorough training in traditional Chinese medicine, may also perform tui-na or be able to provide referrals to practitioners.

TUI-NA TECHNIQUES

In general, tui-na is a fairly vigorous form of massage that employs a variety of hand techniques, usually used in combination.

* *Ma:* Rubbing with the palm or fingertips
* *Pai:* Tapping with the palm or fingertips
* *Ta:* Pinching with thumb and forefinger
* *An:* Rapid, rhythmic pressing with the thumb, palm, or back of the hand
* *Nie:* Grasping an area, then twisting it with fingers and thumbs

CONDITIONS

Although the traditions and practices that fall under touch therapy are diverse, most share a common principle that sets them apart from conventional medicine: health. Following are particular health conditions, each with a range of therapy options—whether acupuncture, Rolfing, or reflexology. Within these profiles, you'll find specific treatment suggestions from the different schools of thought. Explore the wide variety of touch therapies that are available to soothe those conditions that ail you.

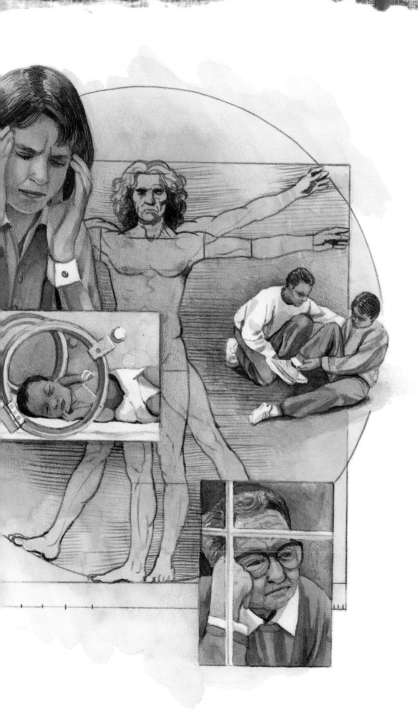

AIDS

Acquired immunodeficiency syndrome, or AIDS, is caused by infection with the human immunodeficiency virus, or HIV. This virus weakens the immune system by inhibiting the production of white blood cells called *T cells*, which fight bacteria and viruses. It is estimated that well over a million Americans are infected with HIV. In the United States, AIDS was first diagnosed in homosexual and bisexual men in the early 1980s; today, heterosexual women are the fastest-growing HIV-infected population.

HIV is spread through contact with infected bodily fluids, mainly semen and blood. The most common means of transmission are anal, oral, and vaginal sex and the sharing of infected hypodermic needles among intravenous-drug users.

A person can be infected with HIV for many years before developing any symptoms. AIDS is likely to appear first as flulike symptoms and weight loss. These are followed by a variety of illnesses, typically Kaposi sarcoma (a type of skin cancer), *Pneumocystis carinii* pneumonia, or tuberculosis. It is not actually AIDS that causes death but other diseases and opportunistic infections that the weakened immune system cannot fight off.

CONVENTIONAL TREATMENT

There is no cure for AIDS. Standard therapy involves potent antiviral drugs, which can prevent the disease from developing, at least temporarily. Currently, doctors are experiencing great success with a regimen that combines several different antivirals. However, the medications are very expensive and must be taken on an exact schedule; failing to do so can cause the virus to become stronger than it was before.

TOUCH THERAPY

HIV infection and AIDS are life-threatening conditions that require medical attention. Alternative treatments should be used only as an adjunct to, never a replacement for, conventional care.

Touch for Mutual Support

There is no cure for AIDS yet, but people with HIV infection and AIDS are living longer thanks in large part to the partial success of newer drugs. But the increased life expectancy does not necessarily increase the HIV-positive person's life certainty—the disease is still incurable and fatal. To counteract the physical, mental, and social effects of their health situation, many people have turned to support groups—gatherings of similarly affected people coming together to share their experiences and wisdom. Increasingly, AIDS/HIV support groups have been incorporating touch therapy into their offerings. Therapeutic Touch, for example, has found a place in many AIDS/HIV groups because it can be quickly taught and members can then administer therapy to each other. Certain Swedish massage techniques can also be administered by properly trained laypeople, and these, too, have a place in this setting.

The Carl Vogel Center in Washington, D.C., has produced a video documenting massage therapy that is complementary to other treatments for HIV/AIDS. The video is available from the Carl Vogel Center at 202-638-0750.

Aromatherapy Massage

Various scents may ease some of the side effects of HIV infection and AIDS, including lemon for anxiety, chamomile and ginger for chronic pain, and bergamot and lavender for depression.

Massage

Research at the Touch Research Institute shows that massage therapy increases immune function in HIV-infected patients. Subjects received 45-minute massages five days a week for a month. Compared with the control period, when they did not receive massage, patients experienced a rise in the number of natural killer cells (a vital indicator of immune function). Patients also had lower levels of cortisol, a stress hormone, and they reported feeling less anxiety.

Therapeutic Touch

Research indicates that Therapeutic Touch reduces the effects of stress on the immune system, which may be beneficial for HIV and AIDS patients.

ANXIETY

Most of us feel a little anxious at some point in our lives. A mildly uneasy feeling can even be beneficial when it helps improve performance. But anxiety becomes a problem when it causes strong feelings of impending doom with no apparent cause. It can inhibit a person's thoughts, disrupt normal daily activities, and cause a host of physical and emotional symptoms.

People with anxiety cannot escape the feeling that something bad is going to happen to themselves or loved ones. They often fear that they are going to lose control, which leads to fatigue, irritability, and an unhealthy dependence on other people. They may also have a strange feeling of being cut off from themselves or from the rest of the world. Symptoms are sometimes so severe that victims of anxiety can become totally disabled.

According to the American Psychiatric Association, "anxiety disorders" refers to a group of illnesses: phobias, panic disorders, post-traumatic stress disorder, and obsessive-compulsive disorders. When people suffering from anxiety disorders talk about their condition, they often refer to these descriptions:

* heart palpitations
* hyperventilation
* insomnia
* gastrointestinal problems, such as diarrhea, nausea, and poor appetite
* light-headedness
* excessive perspiration ("sweaty palms")
* muscle tension, particularly in the neck and shoulders
* trembling
* dry mouth

Several theories exist to explain the cause of anxiety:

* Research has shown that anxious people experience a heightened state of arousal in their central nervous systems. This creates overexcited reactions to life events, which sets off a vicious cycle: Over-reaction leads to physical symptoms of anxiety, which, in turn, reinforces feelings of anxiety.

- Freudian-based theory contends that anxiety is caused by unresolved childhood experiences that have been repressed.
- According to behavioral psychology, anxiety is a learned response. Originally experienced as a performance enhancer, anxiety becomes a conditioned response to even minor problems.

CONVENTIONAL TREATMENT

Psychotherapy is typically recommended for anxiety disorders. Medications may also be prescribed. Sometimes a combination of psychotherapy and medication is recommended:

- Benzodiazepine drugs—a type of tranquilizer—reduce nerve activity in the brain and temporarily create a state of relaxation but can be habit forming and may cause drowsiness and confusion.
- Beta-blockers—drugs sometimes prescribed for high blood pressure—ease physical symptoms such as shaking and palpitations.
- Antidepressants, although often helpful, can cause mouth dryness, dizziness, and blurred vision.

MEDITATION MADE EASY

Though it may have New Age overtones, meditation is actually a well-researched discipline proven to reduce anxiety levels. Meditation induces the relaxation response. Meditation is not difficult to learn, and just 20 minutes a day can be beneficial.

- Choose a quiet place and eliminate distractions. Turn off the telephone and ask others in your household not to disturb you.
- Sit in a comfortable position where you can remain for the entire period with your spine erect. Many people sit cross-legged on the floor, but sitting in a chair is fine too.
- Close your eyes and pick a focal point. This can be a single word (such as "peace" or "calm"), a peaceful image (such as a burning candle or placid lake), or simply a count of your breaths ("one" on the in breath, "two" on the out breath). Repeat or hold the focal point in your mind for 20 minutes.
- When your mind wanders, gently bring it back to the chosen focal point. Do not become upset with yourself. Remember, the only definition of a good meditation is that you did it.

TOUCH THERAPY

Aromatherapy Massage

A variety of scents are reputed to reduce anxiety. Among the most effective:

- lavender
- marjoram
- lemon
- bergamot
- sandalwood

Jin Shin Jyutsu

The philosophy of this pressure-point technique connects different emotions with each finger. Worry is the domain of the thumb, and pressing it gently until you feel yourself relax may help alleviate anxiety.

Massage

A number of studies have found that massage eases anxiety. Research has shown positive results specifically for reducing anxiety in cancer patients, depressed children and teenagers, women with eating disorders, and fibromyalgia patients. One study found that 30 minutes of massage a day was more effective at alleviating anxiety than a relaxation video.

Massage causes a number of physiologic responses that play a role in reducing anxiety. Among the many benefits, it:

- triggers the release of endorphins, hormones that create a sense of well-being

- reduces muscle tension
- slows heart rate
- lowers blood pressure
- improves digestion
- reduces levels of stress-related hormones
- induces a relaxation response

Reflexology

Practitioners say anxiety may be eased by working on points connected to the diaphragm and the pituitary, thyroid, and adrenal glands.

Rolfing

One study found that after five weeks of Rolfing treatment, subjects experienced a significant decrease in anxiety. The researchers theorize that Rolfing caused a release of emotional tension that had been stored in the muscles, which, in turn, resulted in lower scores on a psychological test of anxiety.

Therapeutic Touch

Research has shown that Therapeutic Touch prompts the relaxation response, a physiologic state in which heart and breathing rates drop, brainwave activity slows, and muscles become less tense. Levels of various body chemicals associated with anxiety and stress also decline.

ARTHRITIS

Arthritis isn't a single disorder but rather a broad term that encompasses several specific types. The two major chronic types are rheumatoid arthritis and osteoarthritis. Unfortunately, in most cases, the disease cannot be stopped completely. However, many types of touch therapy can greatly alleviate the symptoms of arthritis.

Arthritis involves inflammation of one or more joints, which leads to pain, stiffness, swelling, and redness. The different types of arthritis have different causes:

* Rheumatoid arthritis is the most severe form. It is an autoimmune disorder in which the body's immune system attacks and damages joints and surrounding tissue, most commonly in the hands, feet, and arms. It is extremely painful and can cause physical deformity.
* Osteoarthritis is the most common type and is caused by wear and tear on the joints. It tends to appear in middle age, growing worse over time.

Infectious arthritis, an acute form of the disease, is the result of bacteria invading a joint, usually from an infected wound near the joint or because of infection elsewhere in the body. This form of arthritis is typically treated with antibiotics.

Symptoms of arthritis include:

* swelling pain and stiffness in one or more joints
* limited range of motion
* red, hot, and burning skin around the joints (rheumatoid arthritis); pain can be worse after prolonged inactivity in the affected joints.
* increased pain with overuse of the joint (osteoarthritis)

CONVENTIONAL TREATMENT

Aimed at controlling symptoms, standard medical therapy for arthritis usually combines medication, exercise, and, in the case of severe flare-ups, bed rest. Among the drugs commonly prescribed are:

* aspirin to alleviate pain
* nonsteroidal anti-inflammatory drugs, such as ibuprofen

* corticosteroids to reduce inflammation and suppress the immune system (rheumatoid arthritis)

Extremely painful or deformed joints may require surgery to replace the joint with an artificial one or to fuse the bones in the joint to stabilize it.

TOUCH THERAPY

Acupressure

Stimulating various acupressure points may alleviate some of the pain and swelling of arthritis. In particular, Gall Bladder 20 is an anti-inflammatory point that relieves pain all over the body. It is located at the back of the neck in line with the first thoracic vertebrae, two finger widths on either side of the spine.

Chiropractic

Chiropractic treatments may alleviate pain for many arthritis sufferers, particularly in the case of osteoarthritis. Misaligned spinal vertebrae and joints place abnormal stress throughout the body, which can make osteoarthritis worse. Chiropractic adjustment focuses on bringing the spine into proper alignment, which can alleviate pain and restore normal movement.

Craniosacral Therapy

Practitioners say that craniosacral therapy can alleviate arthritis pain.

EAT FOR HEALTH

Proper diet and nutrition are essential to treating arthritis and can help enhance the benefits patients experience from touch therapy. Here are some basics to keep in mind.

* Maintain an ideal body weight. Extra pounds put pressure on the joints, which can exacerbate osteoarthritis in particular.
* Limit animal foods. Research has shown that a vegetarian diet can improve symptoms of rheumatoid arthritis. Certain animal foods, including meat, milk, cheese, and butter, contain a fatty acid that may contribute to inflammation.
* Consume cold-water fish, such as salmon, herring, and sardines. These are especially rich in fatty acids that help control inflammation in rheumatoid arthritis. Flaxseed and evening primrose oil are other good sources.
* Test for food allergies. Wheat, corn, and dairy products are among the most common allergenic foods that can make arthritis worse.

Massage

Research shows that massage reduces muscle tension and prompts the body to release endorphins—natural chemicals that behave like morphine, decreasing pain and producing a feeling of well-being. Massage also has benefits that can be helpful for the emotional aspects of chronic pain: It reduces anxiety and causes the relaxation response.

Massage can reduce swelling around joints, which can reduce stiffness. It also relieves tension in surrounding muscles that may have been affected by the afflicted joint's limited range of motion.

Myofascial Release

Myofascial release can alleviate restrictions in connective tissue that pull muscles and bones out of place, which can contribute to osteoarthritis.

Osteopathic Medicine

Osteopathic manipulation of the joints and soft tissue may help ease pain and increase mobility. Osteopathic physicians can prescribe medication if necessary.

Rolfing

Ida Rolf created her technique of structural integration largely because she sought relief from her own arthritis. Rolfing has helped many osteoarthritis sufferers in particular. Stretching the fascia—the connective tissue that surrounds muscles and connects them to the bones—can alleviate structural abnormalities that strain muscles, tendons, and joints. Realigning the body reduces wear and tear, improving movement and bringing relief from pain.

Physical Therapy

Various techniques of physical therapy can bring relief from pain and restore more movement, especially for osteoarthritis. One of the modalities a physical therapist may use for arthritis pain is hydrotherapy, or treatment with water. Warm, moist heat applied in a compress can help alleviate pain and stiffness. A program of isometric exercises and swimming can help increase circulation to the affected joints and improve muscle strength without stressing the joints.

Therapeutic Touch

Practitioners say Therapeutic Touch can alleviate chronic pain, and research indicates it prompts the relaxation response.

ASTHMA

A serious chronic disease that affects as many as 15 million Americans, asthma causes swelling in the bronchial tubes and difficult breathing. Asthma is more common in children than adults; it may become less severe as a child grows up. In some people, the condition is fairly minor—more of an annoyance than a health risk. For others, however, asthma attacks can be severe enough to be life-threatening and require emergency treatment.

Asthma occurs in two forms: extrinsic and intrinsic. Extrinsic asthma tends to develop earlier in life and is caused mainly by inhaling allergens, such as pollen, dust, animal dander, and mold. Other factors can also cause extrinsic asthma, including:

✿ respiratory infection
✿ exercise, especially in cold air
✿ food or drug allergies
✿ air pollution, especially tobacco smoke

Intrinsic asthma has no apparent cause, though it often makes its first appearance after a respiratory tract infection. Stress and anxiety may also provoke attacks.

During an asthma attack, muscle spasms and swollen breathing tubes cause difficulty inhaling air, which can cause anything from mild breathlessness to respiratory failure. The episode may pass in just a few minutes or may last as long as a day. There is no cure for asthma. Instead, the focus is on controlling asthmatic episodes.

CONVENTIONAL TREATMENT

Because allergies are a primary cause of asthma, allergy testing is a key first step in treatment. Immunotherapy—better known as allergy shots—may then be recommended to help the patient's immune system build up a resistance to any allergens.

Several different types of drugs are used to prevent attacks or control them once they've started:

✿ Inhaled or oral bronchodilator drugs, such as albuterol,

relax and widen the airways, relieving chest tightness and wheezing.

* Corticosteroids may be prescribed in severe cases to ease inflammation in the breathing tubes.
* Epinephrine may be required in an emergency situation to open the airways.

TOUCH THERAPY

Asthma is a serious condition that requires medical attention. Alternative therapies should be used as a supplement to, rather than replacement for, conventional care.

Acupressure

Pressing gently on an acupressure point on the lungs' meridian can help prevent breathing problems and ease them when they do occur. The point, called Lung 1 (or Lu 1), is about a half-inch below the large hollow of collarbone on the outer part of both sides of the chest, on the sensitive spot near the shoulder.

Aromatherapy Massage

As with any serious health condition, asthmatics should not use essential oils without the advice of a qualified health practitioner.

As a preventive measure, the aroma of certain essential oils may help ease respiratory congestion:

* eucalyptus
* German chamomile
* lavender
* frankincense
* rosemary

A variety of scents are reputed to reduce anxiety, which can exacerbate asthma. Among the most effective are:

* lavender
* marjoram
* lemon
* bergamot
* sandalwood
* Roman chamomile

Chiropractic

Misalignment of spinal vertebrae can cause restricted breathing. Chiropractic adjustment corrects the misalignment and may help to ease symptoms.

TRACK OUR TRIGGERS

An asthma attack is often caused by a combination of factors. If a person is feeling relaxed, for instance, mild exposure to dust may not trigger an attack, but if he is feeling anxious or stressed, it may be more likely to cause breathing problems. To help identify the things that trigger attacks, keep a journal noting the environmental and emotional factors present during an asthmatic episode.

Medical Massage

A study at the Touch Research Institute found that massage was beneficial for asthmatic children. The children, most of whom had been hospitalized at least once for asthma, were given 20-minute massages by their parents every night before bedtime for a month. Compared with children with asthma who did not receive massages, the treated children experienced a decrease in anxiety and stress hormones, and their peak air flow and pulmonary functions improved.

Reflexology

Practitioners say anxiety may be eased by working on points connected to the diaphragm and the pituitary, thyroid, and adrenal glands. Massaging zones associated with the respiratory system may also be beneficial.

Rolfing

One study found that after five weeks of Rolfing treatment, subjects experienced a significant decrease in anxiety—a contributing factor in some asthma attacks. The researchers theorize that Rolfing caused a release of emotional tension that had been stored in the muscles, which, in turn, resulted in lower scores on a psychological test of anxiety.

Shiatsu

Research indicates that shiatsu massage may help improve symptoms of asthma.

Therapeutic Touch

Research has shown that Therapeutic Touch prompts the relaxation response—a physiologic state in which heart and breathing rates drop, brainwave activity slows, and muscles become less tense. Levels of various body chemicals associated with anxiety and stress also decline. Studies of hospital patients found that Therapeutic Touch was more effective than simple touch in alleviating anxiety.

AUTISM

Though it is a rare condition, autism can be heartbreaking when it occurs. Affecting approximately 2 to 4 out of every 10,000 children, autism is characterized by an inability to form relationships with other people. Often one of the first symptoms to appear in an autistic child is extreme resistance to being touched.

Autistic children may be normal for the first few months after birth, with symptoms becoming evident by 30 months of age. Among the signs of autism are:

* remaining isolated from others
* violently resisting change: Routines and rituals become extremely important
* delayed or complete lack of speech
* behavioral abnormalities: self-injury, finger-twiddling, and hyperactivity

A definite cause for autism is not known, though experts believe the source is brain damage, given that many patients develop epilepsy by the time they become teenagers.

CONVENTIONAL TREATMENT

There is no cure for autism, though behavioral therapy can sometimes reduce self-injury. Medication may be prescribed to alleviate epileptic seizures or hyperactivity.

TOUCH THERAPY
Craniosacral Therapy

According to some practitioners, craniosacral therapy can reduce antisocial and self-destructive behaviors.

Massage

One small study found that massage reduced autistic behavior in preschool-age children. One group of autistic children received 30 minutes of massage twice a week, and another group played a matching-objects game while being held for a comparable amount of time. After five weeks, the children in the massage group showed improved behavior scores, including socially relating to their teachers more often.

BACK PAIN

One of the most common ailments around, back pain affects 80 percent of Americans at some point in their lives. It's the greatest cause of lost work time and the main source of disability for people under 45. Poor posture, a sedentary lifestyle, and extra pounds can all make you more prone to back problems.

In most cases of back pain, a specific cause isn't known. Possibilities include:

❋ herniated intervertebral disk, the spongy pads that separate the spinal vertebrae (sometimes inaccurately called a "slipped" disk)
❋ strains, which involve stretching or tearing of the muscles
❋ sprains, or injured ligaments

In some cases, these factors can be traced to a single event, such as slipping and falling on a patch of ice or playing basketball without proper conditioning. More often, though, the sudden onset of back pain is actually the result of years of abuse or wear and tear. Slouching at a desk, lifting objects improperly, not getting enough exercise, being overweight, and allowing back and stomach muscles to become weak all cause wear on back muscles,

ligaments, and disks, eventually resulting in pain.

CONVENTIONAL TREATMENT

The traditional advice was to follow bed rest for several days or weeks and take painkillers. However, a few years ago, the U.S. Agency for Health Care Policy and Research issued new guidelines for treating back pain. The report recommends a program of spinal manipulation, light activity, and if necessary, over-the-counter anti-inflammatory medications.

In more serious cases, prescription medications may be recommended, including:

❋ muscle relaxants
❋ corticosteroids to ease inflammation
❋ antidepressants in low doses to help patients sleep
❋ narcotic painkillers, such as codeine

Severe cases may require surgery to alleviate pain caused by nerve damage. However, surgery does not address herniated disks, and many critics contend that back surgery is overperformed.

The best treatment for back pain is to take measures to prevent it:

* Shed extra pounds if you are overweight.
* Exercise regularly.
* Sit up straight, if necessary using a lumbar pillow to preserve the natural curve of the spine.
* Move about regularly throughout the day, getting up to walk around for a few minutes at least once an hour, more if possible.
* Sleep on a firm mattress.

TOUCH THERAPY
Aromatherapy Massage

Many different scents are said to ease muscle pain:

* camphor
* eucalyptus
* lavender
* peppermint
* thyme
* chamomile
* ginger
* marjoram
* rosemary

Chiropractic Medicine

Treating back pain is chiropractic's specialty. Numerous studies, including a report from the U.S. government, have found spinal manipulation to be the safest, most effective therapy for acute back pain. Research also shows that compared with back-pain patients who use standard medical care, chiropractic patients experience greater improvement, lower health care costs, and fewer lost work days; they are also more satisfied with their care.

According to chiropractic theory, misalignment of the vertebrae in the spine can cause the joints to press on spinal nerves, causing pain in the back and other areas of the

YOGA FOR PREVENTION

An excellent yoga exercise for strengthening the lower back is the cat–dog pose, sometimes called the "self-chiropractor." Get down on your hands and knees. Inhale and let your spine drop, curving toward the ground, as you raise your head. Then exhale as you raise your spine into an arch and drop your head down. (Keep your arms straight at all times.) Repeat this movement with each inhalation and exhalation, for one to three minutes a day.

Many cases of back pain eventually clear up on their own without any treatment at all. If, however, you have any of the following symptoms, be sure to see a physician:

* problems controlling your bowels or bladder
* numbness in the groin or rectal area
* extreme leg weakness
* pain continuing for more than two weeks

body. Chiropractors treat back pain by manipulating the vertebrae and joints in the spine, restoring them to their proper positions.

Craniosacral Therapy

Practitioners say that craniosacral therapy can alleviate chronic pain, including back pain. An advanced craniosacral technique called unwinding focuses on releasing specific trauma from the body by recreating the position of the body when the trauma occurred, which may be helpful if back pain is the result of injury.

Massage

Massaging the muscles around the spine can relieve tightness and help improve mobility. Also, massage has been shown to prompt the release of endorphins, natural chemicals that behave like morphine, killing pain and producing a sense of well-being. However, deep-

tissue massage can worsen some serious conditions, including herniated disks.

An episode of intense back pain often involves the spraining of certain muscles that support the spine. These sprains themselves can be quite painful. Massage can reduce back pain caused by such sprains and can facilitate their healing by improving circulation.

Myofascial Release

Myofascial release can alleviate restrictions in connective tissue that pull muscles and bones out of place, which can contribute to back pain.

Osteopathic Medicine

Studies have shown that osteopathic manipulation can decrease recovery time in cases of back pain. Spinal manipulation, including that performed by osteopathic physicians, is among the U.S. government's primary treatment recommendations for back pain. Because osteopaths are qualified to prescribe medication, pharmaceutical treatment is also an option for a DO.

Physical Therapy

Physical therapists are qualified to diagnose and treat problems related to physical function, including back pain. The goal is to help patients regain as much normal physical function as possible. Physical therapists have a wide variety of modalities at their disposal, including:

* joint mobilization
* relaxation exercises
* biofeedback
* electrical stimulation
* hydrotherapy
* traction
* heat
* ultrasound
* ice therapy
* laser therapy
* chiropractic manipulation
* massage

Physical therapy also is beneficial for developing a preventive program of exercise and movement strategies.

Shiatsu

One study found that two weekly shiatsu massages provided significant relief of chronic back pain for the majority of study subjects, many of whom had not responded to mainstream treatment or even acupuncture.

Structural and Functional Techniques

Rolfing and Hellerwork involve deep-tissue and joint manipulation, which can realign the body and decrease structural imbalances that cause back pain. These as well as the other movement re-education therapies also teach patients new patterns of movement that can reduce back pain.

COOL IT NOW

When a "back attack" happens, you may be inclined to apply heat to the area because it feels soothing, but heat can increase swelling if applied too soon. For the first 24 to 48 hours after the onset of pain, apply ice to the painful area to reduce inflammation. After a day or two, use moist heat, such as a wet washcloth or a hot water bottle wrapped in a moist towel, to stimulate blood circulation to the area, which increases the removal of waste products and speeds healing.

BLADDER INFECTIONS

Technically known as cystitis, bladder infections are relatively common in women and very rare in men. That's because a woman's urethra—the tube through which urine passes out of the body—is much shorter, which makes it easier for bacteria to work their way into the bladder. In men, bladder infections nearly always are the result of an obstruction, typically an enlarged prostate that presses on the urethra.

In women, the bacteria that cause bladder infections can come from many sources:

* the anus or vagina, both of which are close to the opening of the urethra
* sexual intercourse, which can push bacteria into the bladder
* use of a diaphragm for birth control, which can press on the bladder and lead to incomplete elimination of urine

Bladder infections usually are not serious if they're treated right away. Recurring infections, however, can can sometimes result in kidney infection, which can be very serious and cause permanent damage.

Several symptoms characterize bladder infections:

* burning or pain during urination
* difficulty urinating
* frequent need to urinate with only a small amount produced
* urine that smells foul
* pain in the lower abdomen or back
* vomiting, nausea, and fever—usually a sign the infection is affecting the kidneys

CONVENTIONAL TREATMENT

Antibiotics are the usual treatment for cystitis. Preventive measures for women who are prone to recurrent infections are also an emphasis; these include:

* drinking large quantities of fluid, including cranberry juice
* urinating whenever you feel the urge and emptying the bladder completely
* emptying the bladder immediately after sex

THE CRANBERRY CURE

Drinking several glasses of cranberry juice each day has long been a home remedy for preventing bladder infections. (It's also used as a treatment, but because it is so acidic, you may find that it increases the burning sensation during urination.) Now scientific research not only documents the benefits of the cranberry cure but also suggests why it is so effective: It seems to prevent bacteria from adhering to the bladder wall. If you don't care for cranberry juice, which tends to contain large amounts of sweetener, the berry also is available as an herbal supplement in capsule or tablet form.

* wiping with toilet tissue from front to back
* wearing cotton underwear to avoid trapping heat and moisture
* avoiding perfumed soaps, bubble bath, and douches

TOUCH THERAPY

Acupressure

Stimulating points along the stomach meridian may help alleviate bladder infections.

Aromatherapy Massage

Several aromas are said to improve healing in the urinary tract:

* eucalyptus
* juniper
* sandalwood
* thyme

Diluted in a light vegetable oil, such as almond oil, these can be massaged over the lower back, abdomen, and stomach on a daily basis.

Chiropractic

Realigning the lower spine may help strengthen the muscles of the bladder and prevent bladder infections.

Osteopathic Medicine

As with chiropractic, realigning the lower spine may help strengthen bladder muscles and prevent bladder infections. (Osteopaths also can prescribe antibiotics to treat an existing bladder infection when necessary.)

Reflexology

Applying pressure to the bladder and kidney zones may help alleviate the pain of bladder infections.

BONE SPURS

Abnormal growth at the end of a bone can lead to bone spurs—knobby growths that can cause sharp, shooting pain. Typically found in the spine and feet, bone spurs usually afflict older people with spinal disk problems, but they can also be a problem for people who tend to put physical stress on their body, such as dancers and waiters.

Spurs can grow on a variety of bones in the foot, but the kind that's most often associated with pain is the heel spur. Because the weight of your whole body presses down on your heel, any pain in that area is intensified.

CONVENTIONAL TREATMENT

Over-the-counter or prescription anti-inflammatory drugs are usually recommended. For bone spurs on the spine, an orthopedic collar may be needed to reduce movement and alleviate pain. For foot spurs, the best temporary relief is to keep from exerting continued pressure on it—by staying off the foot and keeping it out of shoes as much as possible. When you must wear shoes, foam inserts can relieve pressure and pain. Surgery may also be required. A doctor may prescribe weight loss as well.

TOUCH THERAPY
Chiropractic

Chiropractic practitioners believe realigning the spine can

COLD RELIEF

Tactile healing can be expanded to more than human touch. Hydrotherapy involves the use of water and can alleviate the pain of a bone spur. Wrap some ice or an ice pack in a towel and apply it to the painful area for 10 minutes. Then remove for 10 minutes before applying for an additional 10 minutes. Do not exceed 20 minutes total or you may damage the skin. If you feel pain after exercise, apply the cold after the exercise is complete; if you feel pain during and after exercise, apply the cold during and after.

The Healing Power of Touch

help alleviate the wear and tear that leads to bone spurs.

Massage

Deep-tissue massage can reduce restrictions in the fascia, the connective tissue that surrounds all muscles and joins them to the bones. In particular, physical stress can inflame the fascia in the feet, creating irritation that leads to calcification in the bone. Therapy can promote healing and reduce swelling in the plantar fascia that covers the bottom of the feet, especially in the heel, which is a common site for bone spurs.

Myofascial Release

Myofascial release can alleviate restrictions in connective tissue that pull muscles and bones out of place, which can contribute to development of bone spurs.

Osteopathic Medicine

Realigning the spine can help alleviate the wear and tear that leads to bone spurs.

Structural and Functional Techniques

Rolfing and Hellerwork involve deep-tissue massage, which can alleviate restrictions that lead to calcification in the bone. These techniques, as well as the other types of movement re-education, teach patients new patterns of movement to reduce the physical stress that can lead to bone spurs.

BRONCHITIS

Bronchitis is an inflammation of the bronchial tubes—the airways that connect the windpipe to the lungs. Characterized by a persistent cough and copious amounts of phlegm, bronchitis comes in two forms: acute and chronic. Both types are most common in smokers and in people who live in heavily polluted areas.

Acute bronchitis tends to come on suddenly, usually on the heels of a viral infection such as a cold or the flu. (Rarely, bacterial infection is the cause.) It usually occurs during the wintertime. Symptoms include:

* wheezing
* breathlessness
* persistent cough
* yellow or green phlegm
* a feeling of tightness in the chest
* pain behind or below the breastbone
* occasionally a fever

Acute bronchitis tends to clear up in a few days, except in the elderly and those with lung disease, who tend to have lower disease resistance.

Chronic bronchitis is diagnosed when a patient coughs up phlegm on most days during three consecutive months for at least two years in a row.

Cigarette smoking is the main cause of chronic bronchitis, which leads to narrow, obstructed airways in the lungs. Chronic bronchitis often is found in conjunction with emphysema, a condition in which the air sacs in the lungs become distended.

CONVENTIONAL TREATMENT

In acute cases caused by bacterial infection, a physician will prescribe antibiotics; these are also sometimes advised in cases of viral infection, to prevent weakened lungs from succumbing to bacterial infections. Warm steam, from a shower or humidifier, can alleviate symptoms. Drinking plenty of fluids is also recommended to help expectorate the mucus. Cough-suppressant medication is not usually advised unless coughing is interfering with getting adequate rest.

Reflexology may offer some symptomatic relief for those suffering from bronchitis. The lung reflex area, located on the bottoms of the feet, extends from the base of the toes through the balls of the foot. Press the tips of the thumbs into the troughs found between the toe bones in the lung area while you press the tips of the index fingers into the corresponding troughs on the top of the foot.

Patients with chronic bronchitis are urged to quit smoking and, if necessary, to lose weight to avoid straining the heart. They typically require oral or inhaled bronchodilators, which are medications that dilate constricted airways. Bronchodilators can cause heart palpitations and high blood pressure. In severe cases, patients may require an oxygen tank.

TOUCH THERAPY

Though acute bronchitis may resolve on its own, conventional medical care often is necessary, particularly if antibiotics are required. Alternative therapies should be used as a supplement to, rather than replacement for, conventional care.

Aromatherapy Massage

Certain essential oils may help alleviate various symptoms of bronchitis:

* Eucalyptus is an expectorant.
* Tea tree has antiseptic properties.
* Thyme is an antiseptic and expectorant.

Chiropractic and Osteopathic Medicine

Spinal adjustment may help ease breathing restrictions.

Massage

Percussive techniques can help expectorate mucus from the lungs. Massaging the muscles in the neck, shoulders, chest, and back can ease tension and may improve breathing.

Reflexology

Applying pressure to the zones connected to the lungs, solar plexus, and adrenals may help alleviate symptoms of bronchitis (see sidebar, above).

Shiatsu

Research indicates that shiatsu massage can help alleviate bronchitis.

BUNIONS

Associated with weak foot structure, bunions occur when the joint at the base of the big toe is forced outward, creating a fluid-filled sac on the side of the foot—the bunion—which can become inflamed, swollen, and painful. As the joint moves out, the big toe points in, sometimes overlapping the second toe. Often hereditary in nature, bunions can be exacerbated by uncomfortable shoes. Bunions require treatment, or they will become progressively worse.

CONVENTIONAL TREATMENT

Over-the-counter or prescription anti-inflammatory pain medication is typically recommended for minor bunion pain. Although bunion pads are readily available, they can end up creating pressure in other parts of the foot, so orthotics—specially made shoe inserts that relieve pressure—are usually preferred. Surgery is sometimes recommended but may not provide permanent relief.

TOUCH THERAPY

Chiropractic and Osteopathic Medicine

Spinal or leg adjustments can alleviate structural imbalances that can lead to bunions.

Massage

Foot massage can help alleviate discomfort and reduce swelling.

Structural and Functional Techniques

Rolfing and Hellerwork involve deep-tissue massage, which can alleviate restrictions that lead to misalignment of the joint. These techniques, as well as the other types of movement re-education, also teach patients new patterns of movement to reduce the physical stress that can lead to bunions.

Easing the Pain

* A hot footbath can ease the pain and inflammation associated with the condition.
* Topical analgesic creams with capsaicin—the natural chemical that gives chili peppers their zing—can also help reduce pain and inflammation.
* Going barefoot as often as possible reduces restrictions on the feet that exacerbate bunions.

BURNS

Skin is living tissue, and exposure to heat can damage it. Two million people are burned in the United States each year, many of them seriously enough to require hospitalization. Most burns are the result of household accidents, and children and the elderly are the most common victims.

Burns have three different stages of severity:

* First-degree burns affect only the top layer of skin, causing it to redden (as in the case of sunburn) without blisters. Most minor sunburns and kitchen burns are first degree. Although they can be painful, first-degree burns tend to heal fairly rapidly.

* Second-degree burns cause deeper damage and blisters. Unless they are large or become infected, these too tend to heal fairly quickly, usually without scarring.

* Third-degree burns are extremely serious and destroy all layers of skin, leaving it charred or waxy in appearance.

CONVENTIONAL TREATMENT

First-degree and minor second-degree burns may involve pain, headache, and fever; they are treated with analgesics such as aspirin and acetaminophen.

Second-degree and third-degree burns covering more than 10 percent of the body leave the victim in shock and require hospitalization. Third-degree burns can be fatal if they cover a large area. Intravenous fluids, antibiotics, antibacterial dressing, and plastic surgery are standard treatments for these more extensive injuries.

TOUCH THERAPY

Serious burns require medical care. Alternative therapies should be used as a supplement to, rather than replacement for, conventional care.

Aromatherapy Massage

Lavender oil may speed healing in minor burns.

Massage

Massage has been shown to reduce levels of cortisol—a

FIRST AID FOR MINOR BURNS

First-degree burns, minor second-degree burns, and sunburn all can be treated with home remedies; more serious burns require medical attention.

Immerse minor burns in cool water for 10 minutes, or run cool water over them to reduce the temperature. Keep the area clean and apply a sterile dressing. Or apply fresh aloe vera juice, which research has shown to reduce skin damage from burns and speed healing. (Keep a plant in a sunny window for household emergencies.) Cut open one of the plant's fleshy leaves and squeeze out the juice onto the burn, then leave the area uncovered.

Lavender essential oil is another excellent remedy for minor burns. In fact, the chemist who became known as the father of modern aromatherapy decided to devote his life to the healing art after he burned his hand in a lab accident, stuck it in a vat of lavender oil, and was astonished by its rapid healing power. Before applying lavender oil, dilute two or three drops in a tablespoon or two of aloe vera juice or water.

Never apply butter or any other greasy, oily, or fluffy dressing on a burn. These fatty substances hold heat in and slow down healing. Also, such substances increase the risk of infection.

stress hormone—in burn patients. Research also has found that massage reduces burn patients' anxiety, improves clinical symptoms, and decreases recovery time. Other research has found that massage prompts the release of endorphins, the body's natural painkillers. Certain massage techniques may also soften the scarring that can follow a burn.

Therapeutic Touch

Therapeutic Touch has been shown to speed wound healing, which may have implications for burn patients.

BURSITIS

Bursitis is inflammation in a bursa—the fluid-filled sacs that cushion pressure points in the body, mainly the joints, and reduce friction between body parts. If the bursa are healthy, they make movement easier. If they are injured, they become overfilled with fluid, causing pain and swelling. Overuse, injury, or prolonged pressure on a bursa can cause it to become inflamed, creating pressure on surrounding areas. Chronic bursitis can cause calcification of soft tissue and can permanently impair joint movement.

Bursitis tends to affect joints in the shoulders, elbows, and knees. Some types of bursitis have highly descriptive names:

* *Housemaid's knee* is caused by prolonged kneeling on a hard surface.
* *Frozen shoulder* is sometimes caused by untreated bursitis in the shoulder.
* *Student's elbow* is caused by prolonged pressure against the elbow point from a desk or table.

Bursitis is common in:

* athletes
* people who engage in heavy physical labor
* people whose work involves repetitive motion
* sedentary people who engage in physical activity without proper conditioning

CONVENTIONAL TREATMENT

In severe cases of bursitis, the lining of the inflamed bursa may have to be surgically removed, but most cases are managed with simple rest, ice packs, and over-the-counter anti-inflammatory pain medication. Other conventional treatments for bursitis may include:

* narcotic analgesics, such as codeine
* local injection of cortico-steroids
* antibiotics if infection is present

TOUCH THERAPY
Applied Kinesiology

Applied kinesiologists can help alleviate structural imbalances that create bursitis.

Aromatherapy Massage

Essential oil of lavender is said to alleviate inflammation in soft tissue. However, do not massage it directly on an inflamed bursa; focus instead on the surrounding area.

Chiropractic

Chiropractic adjustments can benefit most musculoskeletal problems, including bursitis. Manipulation can decrease pressure on the inflamed bursa and restore proper alignment and range of motion, which can also ward off future bouts.

Massage

Although massage right on the affected area can actually cause more harm than good, massage of the surrounding tissues can alleviate tension and ease the pain of an inflamed bursa.

Myofascial Release

Myofascial release can alleviate the restrictions in connective tissue that pull muscles and bones out of place and may contribute to bursitis.

Osteopathic Medicine

Like chiropractic adjustments, osteopathic manipulation can benefit most musculoskeletal problems, including bursitis. Manipulation can decrease pressure on the inflamed bursa and restore proper alignment and range of motion, which can prevent further attacks.

Reflexology

Massaging the zone that corresponds to the area where a bursa is inflamed may provide relief.

Structural and Functional Techniques

The deep-tissue massage of Rolfing and Hellerwork can reduce tension around an affected bursa. These, as well as other movement re-education therapies, can teach patients new patterns of movement that alleviate and prevent bursitis.

CANCER

Although there are more than 100 different types of cancer, they all stem from the same fundamental cause: mutated cells that grow uncontrollably. Tumors form when these cells cluster together and continue to spread, depleting the body's tissues of nutrients and destroying healthy cells. Cancerous cells can migrate to other parts of the body through the bloodstream and lymphatic system, forming new, secondary tumors.

Cancer is most common in the major organs, including the lungs, breasts, skin, and stomach. Cancer also can develop in the bone marrow, the lymphatic system, the muscles, and the bones themselves.

Cancer very rarely is caused by any single factor. Instead, it is usually the combined result of numerous risk factors that increase the likelihood of developing the disease. Genetic predisposition and external factors—most commonly smoking, sun exposure, exposure to toxins, and poor diet—are the primary risk factors.

CONVENTIONAL TREATMENT

Today, there are three standard approaches to treating cancer:

* Radiation uses X rays or other types of radiation treatment to reduce tumors prior to surgery, to destroy cancerous cells in a particular part of the body, or to kill cancerous cells that have spread.
* Surgery removes tumors.
* Chemotherapy relies on drugs to eliminate cancerous cells that have spread throughout the body.

All of these approaches are very invasive and can have severe side effects. Radiation and chemotherapy can cause nausea, vomiting, mouth sores, hair loss, and heightened risk of infection. However, given that cancer left untreated is fatal, receiving conventional therapy is critical.

TOUCH THERAPY

Rather than purporting to cure cancer, touch therapy is aimed at relieving various cancer symptoms and side effects of treatment, particularly chronic pain, nausea, anxiety, and stress. Cancer is a serious condition that requires medical attention. Alternative treatments should be used only as an adjunct to, never a replacement for, conventional care.

Acupressure

Stimulating the point called Pericardium 6 has been shown to alleviate nausea and vomiting caused by chemotherapy. Pericardium 6 is located on the inner arm two finger widths above the wrist crease. Acupressure may also ease chronic pain. It is easy to self-administer, but it may be helpful to visit a practitioner to learn which points are best suited for specific pain.

Aromatherapy Massage

One study found that the aroma of Roman chamomile reduced anxiety, tension, and physical symptoms and improved quality of life for cancer patients. Basil essential oil is reputed to alleviate nausea caused by radiation and chemotherapy.

Many different scents are said to ease muscle pain, including:

* camphor
* chamomile
* eucalyptus
* ginger
* lavender
* marjoram
* peppermint
* rosemary
* thyme

Bear in mind that there is much controversy about performing massage on cancer patients, with some experts contending that it may cause cancer to spread. Check with your doctor before receiving massage.

Craniosacral Therapy

Practitioners say that craniosacral therapy can alleviate pain and promote relaxation.

Massage

Research shows that massage reduces muscle tension and alleviates pain. It prompts the body to release endorphins, natural chemicals that behave like morphine, decreasing pain and producing a feeling of well-being. Massage also has benefits that can be helpful for the emotional aspects of cancer. It reduces anxiety and causes the relaxation response, a constellation of physiologic changes that lead to a profoundly relaxed state.

Again, there is much controversy about performing massage on cancer patients, with

ADOPT A HEALTHFUL LIFESTYLE

A number of lifestyle factors can help prevent cancer:

❊ Don't smoke. Smoking is tied to several kinds of cancer, including that of the lungs, bladder, and cervix.

❊ Avoid going into the sun without sunblock.

❊ Exercise regularly. Research shows that sedentary people are much more likely to get cancer than those who exercise.

❊ Eat a low-fat diet based on fruits, vegetables, grains, and legumes. Avoid saturated and trans fats, processed meats, smoked foods, and highly salted foods.

❊ Avoid alcohol or drink it only in moderation.

❊ Keep levels of stress as low as possible; it may be linked to cancer.

some experts contending that it may cause cancer to spread. Check with your doctor before receiving massage.

Reflexology

Reflexology may ease various symptoms, such as pain, nausea, and constipation. It is easy to self-administer, but it may be helpful to visit a practitioner to learn which zones are best suited for your specific issues.

Therapeutic Touch

Practitioners say Therapeutic Touch can alleviate chronic pain, and research indicates it prompts the relaxation response, which can be beneficial in easing the anxiety and stress of having cancer. Studies of hospital patients found that Therapeutic Touch was more effective than simple touch in alleviating anxiety.

CARPAL TUNNEL SYNDROME

Carpal tunnel syndrome is an inflammation of the medial nerve that runs from the forearm to the fingers. Characterized by numbness, tingling, and pain in the thumb, index, and middle fingers, it results from pressure on the nerve that passes through a gap called the carpal tunnel, which is under a ligament at the front of the wrist.

Carpal tunnel syndrome can be caused by a tumor or fracture, but it is more commonly caused by occupations that involve repetitive movements of the hands, especially grasping, turning, and twisting. It often affects middle-aged women, women who are pregnant or just starting birth-control pills, women with PMS, and men and women with underactive thyroids.

CONVENTIONAL TREATMENT

Resting the wrist in a splint may alleviate the problem. Medication such as anti-inflammatories may be recommended to ease pain and inflammation. Injected corticosteroids can also reduce inflammation but have many side effects. In severe cases, surgery is recommended to cut the wrist ligament and ease pressure on the nerve. However, the procedure is not always successful.

TOUCH THERAPY

Acupressure

Pressing points P7, located on the inner wrist in the middle of the crease, and TW4, on the outer wrist at the hollow in the center, for several minutes at a time may relieve pain.

Chiropractic Medicine

Chiropractic manipulation is aimed at easing pressure on the nerve, alleviating pain, and restoring normal function.

Massage

Massage may be beneficial in cases that are exacerbated by muscle tension. It may also reduce the tension surrounding the wrist. Massage of the arms and shoulder can help.

Osteopathic Medicine

Research shows that osteopathic manipulation can help

restore normal function in carpal tunnel syndrome.

Physical Therapy

Physical therapy may use a variety of techniques for treating carpal tunnel syndrome, including:

* deep-tissue massage
* electrical stimulation
* ultrasound
* stretching
* range-of-motion exercises

The goal is to alleviate pain, inflammation, and tension; improve movement of the wrist; and prevent recurrence of carpal tunnel syndrome.

Shiatsu

Shiatsu massage of the forearms may alleviate tension and pain. Ask a practitioner to show you techniques you can use yourself to ease symptoms of carpal tunnel syndrome.

Structural and Functional Techniques

Practitioners of the Alexander Technique report success in alleviating repetitive stress injuries. With their emphasis on training patients to move in ways that reduce physical strain, it's likely that other types of movement re-education also can help treat and prevent carpal tunnel syndrome.

In particular, Aston-Patterning emphasizes ergonomic training, which teaches clients how to restructure their home and work environments to alleviate physical strain. For instance, a patient with carpal tunnel syndrome may be helped by changing the height of her desk chair and using a wrist pad with her computer keyboard.

Hydrotherapy for Self-Help

Applying cold water can ease the pain and inflammation of carpal tunnel syndrome. You can use a cold, wet washcloth, an icepack, or basin of cold water. Do not apply ice for more than 20 minutes, however, because it can damage the skin.

CORRECT DIETARY DEFICIENCIES

A number of studies have found that carpal tunnel syndrome patients tend to be deficient in vitamin B_6. Taking a daily supplement may ease a variety of symptoms, including tingling and numbness. Keep in mind that this remedy can take a couple of months to be effective.

CHRONIC FATIGUE SYNDROME

Going beyond ordinary tiredness, chronic fatigue syndrome is severe, disabling exhaustion accompanied by pain in the joints and muscles. It can last for many months or even several years. The cause of chronic fatigue syndrome is unknown, but it often appears suddenly after a viral infection, possibly implicating an infectious agent.

The disorder appears to have a mind/body connection. Some of the symptoms that tend to accompany it include:

* headaches
* low-grade fever
* recurrent infections
* depression
* poor concentration
* insomnia

The syndrome tends to affect women and, in many cases, women who are perfectionists and have a hard time relaxing.

CONVENTIONAL TREATMENT

Given that the medical establishment can't agree that chronic fatigue syndrome even exists, there is no standard therapy for it. Psychotherapy often is recommended, along with various medications, including:

* over-the-counter analgesics, such as aspirin and aceta-

minophen, for headaches and muscular and joint pain
* benzodiazepine drugs to alleviate anxiety and insomnia
* antidepressants

TOUCH THERAPY
Acupressure

Applying pressure to the gallbladder points may ease fatigue and depression, as well as stimulate the immune system. These points are on either side of the forehead at about the hairline where the part of the hair would be. There are also gallbladder points along the center line on the head.

Aromatherapy Massage

Various essential oils can alleviate some of the symptoms that tend to accompany chronic fatigue syndrome. Scents that can ease depression include:

* bergamot
* clary sage
* lavender
* chamomile
* geranium
* lemon

Scents that may ease headaches include:

* lavender
* marjoram
* lemon
* Roman chamomile
* bergamot
* sandalwood
* peppermint

For insomnia:

* cedar
* marjoram
* neroli
* sandalwood
* lavender
* melissa
* rose

Scents that can ease muscle pain include:

* peppermint
* eucalyptus
* lavender
* chamomile
* ginger
* rosemary

Craniosacral Therapy

Practitioners say that craniosacral therapy can alleviate headaches and musculoskeletal pain, which tend to accompany chronic fatigue syndrome.

Massage

Massage may be helpful in alleviating some symptoms of chronic fatigue. Research shows that massage reduces muscle tension and alleviates pain. It prompts the body to release endorphins, natural painkillers that decrease pain and produce a feeling of well-being. Massage also has benefits that can be helpful for the emotional aspects of chronic pain. It reduces anxiety and causes the relaxation response, a constellation of physiologic changes that lead to a profoundly relaxed state.

Structural and Functional Techniques

These therapies may be beneficial because they are aimed at alleviating muscle pain and enhancing overall well-being.

Therapeutic Touch

Practitioners say that Therapeutic Touch provides relief from musculoskeletal pain, and research indicates that it reduces the effects of stress on the immune system.

CHRONIC PAIN

Millions of Americans suffer chronic pain from a myriad of causes, including injury, illness, and musculoskeletal problems. Most people with chronic pain—by definition, pain that lasts either episodically or continuously for at least six months—take painkillers, but a majority of these patients say they continue to experience intense pain despite the drugs. A growing number of experts have come to view chronic pain not simply as a symptom of other disorders but as an illness in itself.

Pain can range from mild discomfort to excruciating debility. It can stem from problems with the nerves, muscles, or joints; can take many different forms, including numbness, cramping, swelling, aching, or stabbing; and can be diffuse, local, or radiating.

Chronic pain may have no known cause or it may stem from a specific ailment or condition, including:

* AIDS
* arthritis
* back problems
* cancer
* headaches
* injuries that don't heal properly
* multiple sclerosis
* neuralgia (damage to or irritation of a nerve)
* shingles (nerve infection that causes a painful skin rash)
* ulcers

People's tolerance for pain varies widely, and circumstances surrounding the condition may affect a person's perception of pain's intensity. Not knowing the cause, for instance, can create anxiety that makes the pain worse than if the source were understood.

Chronic pain involves more than just physical symptoms. It can also give rise to emotional problems, including anger, anxiety, and depression. This mind/body interaction creates a downward spiral: Besides making the perception of pain more severe, negative emotions create muscle tension, which can make the actual physical pain worse. They also impede the production of endorphins. To make matters worse, research shows that chronic pain can inhibit the immune system, leaving a person more vulnerable to further illness.

CONVENTIONAL TREATMENT

A variety of medications often are used to control chronic pain:

* analgesics, such as aspirin and acetaminophen
* muscle relaxants
* nonsteroidal anti-inflammatory drugs
* narcotics, such as codeine and morphine

However, medications typically do not provide lasting relief, and patients can become dependent on them, particularly narcotic medications. An alternative is available with pain clinics, which tend to take a multidisciplinary approach to helping patients not only reduce their pain but also cope with the emotional effects of it. Therapies may include counseling, biofeedback, acupuncture, and physical therapy.

TOUCH THERAPY

Acupressure

Acupressure may ease chronic pain. It is easy to self-administer, but it may be helpful to visit a practitioner to learn which points are best suited for specific pain.

Aromatherapy Massage

Many different scents are said to ease muscle pain, including:

* camphor
* eucalyptus
* lavender
* peppermint
* thyme
* chamomile
* ginger
* marjoram
* rosemary

Chiropractic and Osteopathic Medicine

Spinal manipulation and soft-tissue massage can alleviate neck and shoulder pain, headaches, backache, and sciatica.

Craniosacral Therapy

Practitioners say that craniosacral therapy can alleviate headaches, musculoskeletal pain, arthritis, and lingering pain from injury. An advanced craniosacral technique called unwinding focuses on releasing specific trauma from the body by recreating the position of the body when the trauma occurred. Because physical trauma often causes psychological trauma, an unwinding session typically leads to emotional release as well.

Massage

Research shows that massage reduces muscle tension and

Reflexology for Pain

Reflexology may offer a way to alleviate some chronic pain. Although you can perform this treatment on yourself, you may find that having another person do it is more effective and more relaxing.

Using the thumb or fingertips, press into the surface of the soles of the feet. Cover the entire surface, using as much pressure as is tolerable. When you come across a spot that is particularly sensitive, spend a little extra time there before moving on.

alleviates pain. It prompts the body to release endorphins. Massage also has benefits that can be helpful for the emotional aspects of chronic pain. It reduces anxiety and causes the relaxation response, a constellation of physiologic changes that lead to a profoundly relaxed state.

Physical Therapy

Physical therapists are qualified to diagnose and treat problems related to physical function, including chronic pain. The goal is to help patients regain as much normal physical function as possible. Physical therapists have a wide variety of modalities at their disposal, including:

* joint mobilization
* relaxation exercises
* biofeedback
* electrical stimulation
* hydrotherapy
* heat
* ultrasound

Reflexology

Reflexology may ease chronic pain. It is easy to self-administer, but it may be helpful to visit a practitioner to learn which zones are best suited for specific pain.

Structural and Functional Techniques

Rolfing and Hellerwork involve deep-tissue and joint manipulation, which realign the body and decrease structural imbalances that cause pain. These as well as the other movement re-education therapies also teach patients new patterns of movement that can reduce pain.

Therapeutic Touch

Practitioners say Therapeutic Touch can alleviate chronic pain, and research indicates it prompts the relaxation response. Studies found that the therapy was more effective that simple touch in alleviating anxiety.

CIRCULATORY PROBLEMS

Circulatory problems typically are experienced in the legs, often as a result of atherosclerosis, or narrowing of the arteries. Cut off from an adequate blood supply, leg muscles ache, cramp, and fatigue easily. The first sign of circulatory problems tends to be pain during walking that is relieved by resting for a few minutes but that recurs once walking resumes. This symptom is known as intermittent claudication.

Circulatory problems usually develop from a combination of factors, including:

- atherosclerosis
- smoking
- obesity
- diabetes
- sedentary lifestyle
- birth control pills

CONVENTIONAL TREATMENT

Treatment is aimed at the underlying ailment causing the circulatory problems. Lifestyle changes often are necessary, including:

- quitting smoking
- losing weight
- exercising
- improving the diet

Aspirin may be recommended, because it inhibits blood clotting, which can cause inflammation and pain. In severe cases, the surgical procedure called angioplasty may be necessary to widen the arteries and improve blood flow.

TOUCH THERAPY
Aromatherapy Massage

Several oils are said to improve general circulation, including:

- basil
- clove
- marjoram
- rosemary
- thyme

Massage

Various types of massage can be used to stimulate circulation and improve localized blood flow.

Reflexology

Reflexology may improve circulation, particularly because gravity pushes blood down to the feet, where it tends to stagnate, rather than moving back up to the heart.

COLIC

About 10 percent of babies suffer from colic—unexplained crying bouts that last for several hours; these episodes can continue for several weeks in a row. A colicky baby tends to draw up her legs, clench her fists, become red in the face, and sometimes pass gas. Colic is not actually a disease and does not have any lasting adverse effects on the baby.

The cause of colic is not known, though it is thought to be the result of spasm in the intestines. The cause of the spasm is also unknown, but may be created by:

* an underdeveloped digestive system
* allergy to foods the mother has consumed (in breast-feeding babies)
* allergy to soy or to cow's milk (in formula-fed babies)
* overfeeding

CONVENTIONAL TREATMENT

There is no cure for colic, other than waiting it out. It normally ceases by three months of age.

TOUCH THERAPY
Acupressure

Using one finger, gently massage the point called Conception Vessel 12, located halfway between the navel and the bottom of the breastbone, for about 15 to 30 seconds.

Craniosacral Therapy

Some practitioners believe that colic is the result of the trauma of birth. Gentle manipulation of the craniosacral system may ease the misalignment and ease the symptoms of colic.

HOME REMEDIES

* Hold the baby stomach down on your forearm while patting or stroking her back.
* Use motion by walking, rocking, or going for a car ride.
* Provide "white noise" by running a vacuum cleaner or clothes dryer where the baby can hear it.
* Place a warm water bottle wrapped in a blanket on the baby's stomach.

COLITIS

Colitis is an inflammation of the mucous membrane lining the large intestine. It can be a painful condition, causing bloody diarrhea and sometimes fever. It's not known exactly what causes various kinds of colitis, which include ulcerative colitis and Crohn disease. It may be a bacterial or viral infection. Prolonged use of antibiotics has been associated with colitis; they kill beneficial bacteria in the gut and may allow harmful bacteria to take hold, producing toxins that irritate the colon. Finally, in some cases, it may be an autoimmune disorder in which the body attacks its own tissue.

CONVENTIONAL TREATMENT

No cure is available for colitis, though mild cases may respond to rest and dietary therapy. Bed rest is also beneficial. If diarrhea has been severe, intravenous feeding may be recommended to rehydrate the patient and give the colon a break. Various drugs, including sulfasalazine and corticosteroids, can control inflammation and alleviate symptoms. When symptoms don't respond to courses of medication, all or part of the colon and rectum can be surgically removed.

TOUCH THERAPY

Colitis is a serious condition that requires medical supervision. Touch therapy should be used as a complement to, rather than a replacement for, conventional care.

Acupressure

Concentrating on points along the stomach and spleen meridians may help ease colitis. The stomach meridian is about halfway between the side of the body and the navel. The spleen meridian runs in a circle around the navel.

Aromatherapy Massage

A variety of scents are reputed to reduce anxiety and stress, which can make colitis worse. Among the most effective are:

- lavender
- marjoram
- lemon
- bergamot
- sandalwood
- Roman chamomile

RELAX FOR RELIEF

Stress and anxiety can make colitis worse; practicing relaxation techniques can help ease the condition. One way to reduce stress is with progressive relaxation, a systematic process of tensing and releasing muscles. Lie on the floor with your hands by your side, then follow these steps:

* Close your eyes and spend a few moments paying attention to the rhythm of your breath.
* Tense the muscles in your right foot for five to 10 seconds, then release. Tense the muscles in your right calf for five to 10 seconds, then release. Tense the muscles in your right thigh for five to 10 seconds, then release.
* Repeat with left foot, calf, and leg.
* Follow this same procedure to tense and release the right buttock, the stomach, then the right hand and arm.
* Repeat with the left buttock, the stomach, then the left hand and arm.
* Lift your shoulders toward your ears, hold for several seconds, then relax. Gently turn your head from side to side a few times.
* Scrunch up your face for several seconds, then release.
* Feeling relaxed, lie still for a few minutes, focusing again on your breathing.
* Gently wriggle your muscles before slowly getting up.

Massage

Research has found that massage therapy eases psycho-emotional distress in patients with chronic inflammatory bowel diseases, including ulcerative colitis and Crohn disease. Massage reduced the frequency of episodes of pain and disability in these patients.

Massage induces the relaxation response, a physiologic state in which heart and breathing rates drop, brain-wave activity slows, and muscles become less tense. Levels of various body chemicals associated with anxiety and stress also decline.

Reflexology

Massaging the zones connected to the colon, liver, adrenal glands, lower spine, diaphragm, and gallbladder may help ease colitis. Press with the thumb in the area of the soles of the feet from about halfway down the foot to the beginning of the heel. Be sure to do both feet.

Rolfing

One study found that after five weeks of Rolfing treatment, subjects experienced a significant decrease in anxiety, which can exacerbate colitis. The researchers theorize that Rolfing caused a release of emotional tension that had been stored in the muscles, which, in turn, resulted in lower scores on a psychological test of anxiety.

Therapeutic Touch

Research has shown that, like massage, Therapeutic Touch prompts the relaxation response—a physiologic response in which heart and breathing rates drop, brainwave activity slows, and muscles become less tense.

Constipation

Constipation—infrequent or difficult bowel movements—is an extremely common symptom, and Americans spend millions of dollars on laxatives each year. Except for the relatively rare cases in which constipation is a symptom of a more serious underlying disorder—such as diverticular disease—it is harmless, though it can be uncomfortable.

Frequency of bowel movements varies by individual; some people may have three a day, while others may have three a week. Therefore, constipation means different things to different people. Technically, though, a person is considered constipated when he has no bowel movement for three days.

Constipation can have a variety of causes, though the biggest problem is not consuming enough fiber or drinking enough water. The National Cancer Institute recommends that adults eat 25 to 35 grams of fiber a day, yet most people consume only half that amount.

Other causes of constipation include:

* stress
* lack of exercise
* pregnancy
* various medications, including antihistamines, antacids, and codeine
* depression
* vitamin and mineral supplements, including iron and calcium
* overuse of laxatives

CONVENTIONAL TREATMENT

Symptoms of constipation include fewer-than-usual bowel movements, straining, hard stools, and sometimes pain and bleeding in the rectal area. Lifestyle measures usually alleviate most cases of constipation. Doctors advise getting regular exercise, drinking eight glasses of water a day, and consuming a high-fiber diet. People should also adopt regular toilet habits; if necessary, sit on the toilet for a few minutes every day at the same time, even if you don't have the urge to go. Never ignore the need to have a bowel movement. Take time to relax. Tension and stress tend to inhibit the bowels from doing

EAT FOR PREVENTION

A diet of white flour, white rice, white pasta, and processed foods can cause constipation, because these foods all contain virtually no fiber. Instead, concentrate on eating:

* whole-grain breads
* brown rice
* whole-grain cereals
* whole-wheat pasta or pasta made from other grains, such as kamut
* oatmeal
* legumes
* fruits
* vegetables

If you are not used to eating high-fiber foods, add them to your diet slowly. Too rapid an increase can cause gas and bloating. Also, be sure to drink a lot of non-caffeinated fluids, to help your digestive system function smoothly.

Keep in mind that if laxatives are used too frequently, the body can become dependent on them for bowel movements. Instead, try natural laxatives, such as psyllium seeds and prunes.

their work. Finally, try natural laxatives such as prunes, dates, and figs.

Constipation that does not respond to these treatments may be a symptom of a more serious condition, including:

* colorectal cancer
* diabetes
* diverticulitis
* irritable bowel syndrome
* multiple sclerosis

See your doctor if your constipation persists for more than five days, you are unable to pass gas, you bleed during a bowel movement, or you have abdominal cramps or fever.

TOUCH THERAPY
Acupressure

Stimulating various acupressure points may relieve constipation:

* Stomach 36, on the outer side of the shinbone, four finger widths below the kneecap
* Large Intestine 11, located at the outer edge of the elbow crease
* Conception Vessel 6, three finger widths below the navel

When using one of these points, press with one finger or the tip of the thumb for 30 to 60 seconds. Use moderate, but tolerable, pressure.

Aromatherapy Massage

Essential oil of rosemary or black pepper are said to alleviate constipation. Others that may be helpful are:

* camphor
* cinnamon
* fennel
* peppermint

Chiropractic and Osteopathic Medicine

Chiropractic and osteopathic manipulation can ease tension in the lower back, which may contribute to constipation.

Massage

Massage has been found to improve digestion and alleviate anxiety and stress, both of which can exacerbate constipation. A specific technique can be applied to affect the movement of the large intestines, which may relieve constipation; you would need a trained practitioner for this therapy.

Reflexology

Massaging the zones connected to the adrenal glands and digestive system may help ease constipation. Press with the thumb in the area of the soles of the feet from about halfway down the foot to the beginning of the heel. Be sure to do both feet.

DEPRESSION

Most people experience normal feelings of sadness or pessimism at least occasionally. Depression occurs when these feelings become deep and unrelenting, leading to an overwhelming sense of hopelessness and worthlessness and sometimes progressing to thoughts of suicide and death. Depression is the most common psychiatric illness, affecting as many as one-third of the population at some point in their lives.

Depression often occurs for no apparent cause, though it can be triggered by such events as the death of a friend or relative, loss of a job, or financial problems. It also can be the result of chemical imbalance in the brain.

Depending on the symptoms, depression can be mild to severe. In mild cases, a person tends to exhibit anxiety and mood swings, sometimes with bouts of crying for no reason. More serious cases include:

* loss of appetite
* insomnia
* lack of interest in activities that were previously enjoyed
* loss of sexual desire
* fatigue
* restlessness
* inability to concentrate

People who suffer serious depression say they feel their lives are pointless. They feel slowed down and useless. Some may even lack the energy to move about or eat. Some depressed patients may have suicidal tendencies.

According to the American Psychiatric Association, some individuals suffer from manic-depressive disorder. Their mood may episodically swing from depression to an abnormal elation or mania that is characterized by hyperactivity, flight of ideas, distractibility, and excessive involvement in activities that often result in painful consequences, such as foolish business investments and reckless driving.

CONVENTIONAL TREATMENT

Although depression can be debilitating, the prognosis is

usually positive, as long as a patient receives appropriate treatment. Psychotherapy is recommended, either in a one-on-one setting or a group. A variety of antidepressant drugs are available to treat chemical imbalances in the brain. Typically, they must be taken for several weeks before they become beneficial, and, in many cases, trial-and-error is needed to find the right medication. Treatment with antidepressants usually lasts for 6 to 12 months. The three main types of antidepressants are:

* tricyclics, such as desipramine and imipramine
* monoamine oxidase (MAO) inhibitors, including phenelzine and tranylcypromine
* serotonin reuptake inhibitors, such as the brand-name drug Prozac

Antidepressants can have a variety of unpleasant side effects, including:

* blurred vision
* blood pressure that drops upon rising from a sitting or lying position
* impotence
* insomnia

In very severe and intractable cases, usually those involving hallucinations, electroconvulsive therapy may be used; this involves applying an electric current to the head.

TOUCH THERAPY

Depression is a serious illness that requires medical care. Alternative therapies should be used as a complement to, rather than replacement for, conventional care.

Aromatherapy Massage

Many essential oils are reputed to uplift the spirits and alleviate depression:

* bergamot
* clary sage
* lavender
* peppermint
* chamomile
* geranium
* lemon

Massage

A number of studies have found that massage eases anxiety and depression. One study found that 30 minutes of massage a day was more effective at alleviating anxiety than a relaxation video. Massage causes a number of physiologic responses that play a role in reducing both anxiety and depression:

* triggers the release of endorphins, hormones that create a sense of comfort and well-being
* reduces muscle tension

WORK OUT, FEEL BETTER

Exercises can help lessen depression by elevating mood and alleviating stress. Research has found that a half-hour of aerobic exercise several times a week can be as effective as counseling for treating depression.

* slows heart rate
* lowers blood pressure
* improves digestion
* reduces levels of stress-related hormones

Research has shown positive results for reducing depression in children and teenagers, women with eating disorders, and fibromyalgia patients.

Rolfing

One study found that after five weeks of Rolfing treatment, subjects experienced a significant decrease in anxiety, which often is a symptom of depression. The researchers theorize that Rolfing caused a release of emotional tension that had been stored in the muscles, which in turn resulted in lower scores on a psychological test of anxiety. The effect of emotional release has been noted in other massage techniques as well.

DIABETES

Diabetes is a condition in which the pancreas produces too little or no insulin. Insulin is a hormone that helps the body's cells absorb glucose, the main source of energy. Without enough insulin to process the glucose, blood levels of glucose become abnormally high. If not controlled, diabetes can lead to a variety of serious health problems and even death.

Diabetes falls into two main categories: type I and type II. Type I, also known as insulin-dependent diabetes or juvenile diabetes, is the more severe form and is caused by insufficient amounts of insulin. It develops quickly, usually affecting children between the ages of 10 and 16. The patient must receive regular injections of insulin or he will fall into a coma and eventually die.

Type II diabetes, also called non-insulin-dependent or adult-onset diabetes, tends to happen gradually and usually affects people over 40. In these patients, the body produces insulin but isn't able to use it effectively. Far more common than type I, type II accounts for about 90 percent of diabetes cases.

Diabetes tends to run in families, though most people who inherit the gene for the condition do not develop it. Type II diabetes seems to be strongly linked to obesity. Other factors that may lead to diabetes, if not directly cause it, include:

* pancreatitis
* infection
* certain medications
* pregnancy (which can lead to temporary diabetes)

The complications of diabetes can be severe. People with type I diabetes who do not take insulin will die, and even people with type II diabetes have a high risk of developing:

* eye problems, including blindness
* damage to the nerves
* kidney damage
* ulcers on the feet, which can lead to gangrene
* atherosclerosis, or narrowing of the arteries
* high blood pressure
* heart attack and stroke

CONVENTIONAL TREATMENT

The goal of diabetes care is to maintain blood levels of glucose that are as normal as possible. For people with type I diabetes, this means regular injections of insulin, as many as four a day. They also must closely regulate their intake of carbohydrates, which the body converts to glucose, to avoid fluctuations of blood glucose levels.

People with type II diabetes often can avoid taking insulin by controlling their diet and weight. Exercise is another important preventive measure, and it can help ward off the cardiovascular effects of diabetes.

TOUCH THERAPY

Diabetes is a serious condition that requires medical attention. Alternative therapies should be used only as an adjunct to, not a replacement for, conventional care.

Massage

A study at the Touch Research Institute found that massage could be beneficial for children with type I diabetes. According to the researchers, nearly a third of diabetic children fail to fully comply with their treatment regimen of insulin therapy, diet control, and exercise; stress has been shown to affect a diabetic child's compliance. In the study, diabetic children received 15-minute massages from their parents before bedtime for a month. They showed decreased levels of stress hormone, improved compliance with insulin and dietary treatment, and lowered levels of blood glucose.

Reflexology

A study at Beijing Medical University found that 30 days of foot reflexology sessions reduced blood glucose levels in patients with type II diabetes.

DIVERTICULAR DISEASE

Diverticular disease can affect any part of the intestines but tends to affect the colon, or lower part of the large intestines. It is characterized by small sacs—called diverticula—that protrude from the inner lining of the intestine. Diverticular disease occurs in two stages: Diverticulosis is the less serious and simply means that diverticula are present. Patients may not even have any sign that they have the condition. Diverticulitis is a complication that occurs when the diverticula become inflamed because of an infection, an obstruction, or even a perforation.

People with diverticulosis may feel cramping on the left side that is alleviated with a bowel movement or passing gas. Sometimes blood may appear in the stools.

Diverticulitis is much more serious. The cramping can feel like appendicitis, except that it's on the left rather than the right side, and it can lead to fever, diarrhea or constipation, pain, tenderness, and a rigid abdomen. In acute diverticulitis, severe attacks occur and then disappear. With chronic diverticulitis, attacks may subside but never completely go away. Left untreated, diverticulitis may lead to abscesses and infection in the diverticula or bowel obstruction.

CONVENTIONAL TREATMENT

A low-fiber diet clearly is a factor in diverticular disease, which is rarely seen in developing countries but is common in the United States and Europe. In cases of diverticulosis, a high-fiber diet often is enough to ward off the disease.

For diverticulitis, bed rest, antibiotics for any infection, and a temporary liquid diet can be sufficient to treat the disease. More severe cases may require hospitalization for intravenous antibiotic treatment and feeding. Surgery may be necessary.

TOUCH THERAPY

Diverticular disease is a serious condition that requires medical supervision. Touch therapy

HIGH-FIBER DIET

A diet of white flour, white rice, white pasta, and processed foods can make you more prone to diverticular disease because they're low in fiber and lead to constipation. Instead, concentrate on eating:

* whole grain breads
* brown rice
* whole grain cereals
* whole wheat pasta or pasta made from other grains, such as kamut
* oatmeal
* legumes
* fruits
* vegetables

If laxatives are used too frequently, the body can become dependent on them for bowel movements. Instead, try natural laxatives, such as psyllium seeds and prunes.

If you are not used to eating high-fiber foods, add them to your diet slowly. Too rapid an increase can cause gas and bloating. Also, be sure to drink a lot of non-caffeinated fluids, to help your digestive system function smoothly.

---

should be used as a complement to, rather than a replacement for, conventional care.

Massage

Because diverticular disease can be stressful, massage may be beneficial. It induces the relaxation response, a physiologic state in which heart and breathing rates drop, brain-wave activity slows, and muscles become less tense. Levels of various body chemicals associated with anxiety and stress also decline. Massage has also been found to improve digestion. Direct massage of the abdominal area followed by drinking a cup of chamomile tea can promote relaxation and allevi-

ate discomfort. Ask your massage therapist how to perform a self-massage of the colon.

Therapeutic Touch

Research has shown that, like massage, Therapeutic Touch prompts the relaxation response, which may be beneficial.

Reflexology

Massaging the zones connected to the adrenal glands, intestines, and solar plexus may be helpful in stimulating digestion and easing inflammation. Press with the thumb in the area of the soles of the feet from about halfway down the foot to the beginning of the heel. Be sure to do both feet.

EPILEPSY

Epilepsy is a neurologic disorder characterized by the repeated occurrence of seizures, which are the result of abnormal electrical activity in the brain. Approximately 1 out of every 200 persons suffers from epilepsy, which can have no apparent cause or may stem from one of many underlying reasons, including genetic predisposition, birth trauma, head injury, brain infection, stroke, and drug or alcohol use.

Epileptic seizures fall into two groups, partial and generalized. Partial seizures stem from a somewhat limited area of the brain and do not necessarily involve unconsciousness. Generalized seizures originate in a large area of the brain, affect the whole body, and cause unconsciousness. Generalized seizures can be further categorized as petit mal seizures, which tend to involve immobility and staring and can happen many times a day, or grand mal seizures, which are much more severe in their symptoms, with the sufferer typically falling, losing consciousness, and jerking about.

CONVENTIONAL TREATMENT

Medication can often reduce the occurrence and severity of epileptic seizures and sometimes stop them altogether.

TOUCH THERAPY

Epilepsy is a serious condition that requires medical attention. Alternative therapies should be used only as an adjunct to, never a replacement for, conventional care.

Craniosacral Therapy

Practitioners have found that aligning the craniosacral system is beneficial for many neurologic conditions, including epileptic seizures. It may be especially helpful for epilepsy caused by birth trauma or injury.

Massage

Stress can bring on epileptic seizures. Because massage has been proven to alleviate stress, it may be helpful in reducing epileptic episodes.

FIBROMYALGIA

Fibromyalgia is a rather mysterious disorder characterized by chronic, generalized muscle pain and stiffness that has no apparent cause. It typically affects the shoulders, back, and hips and tends to appear with a host of other problems, including anxiety, chronic fatigue syndrome, depression, headaches, insomnia, and irritable bowel syndrome.

Fibromyalgia is fairly common, affecting an estimated 5 million Americans and accounting for $60 billion in medical costs each year. The vast majority of fibromyalgia sufferers are women.

CONVENTIONAL TREATMENT

Fibromyalgia is not very well understood, and patients often have been dismissed as hypochondriacs—despite clear evidence of the autoimmune nature of their disease. A rheumatologist may be the most likely specialist to see for fibromyalgia. Various medications may be used, though success is limited:

* analgesics, such as aspirin and acetaminophen
* antidepressants
* anesthetic, such as corticosteroids, injected locally in painful areas

TOUCH THERAPY
Aromatherapy Massage

Many different scents are said to ease muscle pain:

* camphor
* chamomile
* eucalyptus
* ginger
* lavender
* marjoram
* peppermint
* rosemary
* thyme

Essential oils that treat various conditions associated with fibromyalgia may be beneficial. For anxiety and depression:

* bergamot
* chamomile
* lavender
* lemon

For insomnia:

* cedar
* lavender
* marjoram

- melissa
- neroli
- rose
- sandalwood

Massage

A study at the Touch Research Institute found that massage can alleviate various symptoms of fibromyalgia. Patients received 30-minute massages twice a week for five weeks. At the end of the study, patients reported:

- reduced pain and stiffness
- less fatigue
- decreased depression
- less difficulty sleeping

Myofascial Release

Practitioners of myofascial release say it can be very beneficial in alleviating conditions involving chronic pain, including fibromyalgia.

Physical Therapy

Electrical stimulation may be helpful in alleviating muscle pain. Hydrotherapy may also be temporarily beneficial, including ice packs and hot and cold compresses.

Rolfing

Rolfing emphasizes deep-tissue massage, which may be helpful in alleviating the chronic muscular pain of conditions such as fibromyalgia.

Therapeutic Touch

Practitioners say Therapeutic Touch can alleviate chronic pain, and research indicates it prompts the relaxation response. Studies of hospital patients found that Therapeutic Touch was more effective than simple touch in alleviating anxiety.

FOOT PAIN

Foot pain can come from a variety of causes. Some cases are the result of structural problems and wear and tear, whereas others are caused by disease. Sometimes, a specific cause isn't known. Wearing shoes that fit properly—and avoiding high heels—can solve many instances of foot pain.

Different ailments of the foot have different symptoms associated with them:

* Bone spurs are knobby growths that can cause sharp, shooting pain. Bone spurs commonly afflict older people with spinal disk problems, but they can also be a problem for people who tend to put physical stress on their body, such as dancers and waiters (see also page 140).

* Bunions are fluid-filled sacs at the base of the big toe associated with weak foot structure. Bunions cause swelling, inflammation, and pain, as well as restricted movement of the toe joint. Often hereditary in nature, bunions can be exacerbated by uncomfortable shoes. Bunions must be treated or they will become progressively worse (see also page 144).

* Gout is caused by high blood levels of uric acid, which forms crystals, mainly in the big toe but other joints as well. These crystals cause inflammation, pressure, and severe pain. A number of conditions seem to be associated with gout, but it is especially common in men who are overweight, drink alcohol, and eat rich diets full of organ meats and gravy.

* Osteoarthritis is the result of wear and tear on the joints and causes swelling, pain, and stiffness (see also page 127).

* Plantar fasciitis is an inflammation of the connective tissue in the foot and causes heel pain during walking or running. It tends to occur in people who walk or run a lot.

* Rheumatoid arthritis, an autoimmune disorder in which the body attacks its own tissue, leads to swelling, pain, and warmth in the joints, as well as stiffness and limited range of motion (see also page 127).

MASSAGE FOR TIRED DOGS

If your feet are tired and aching because of overuse, an aromatherapy massage can revive them. Dilute two or three drops of peppermint or juniper essential oil in a tablespoon of light vegetable oil. Sit in a chair and cross your right foot over your left leg. Dip your thumb in the oil, then stroke it across the sole of your foot from heel to toe several times, starting in the middle of the foot, then doing the left and right sides. Repeat, but this time instead of stroking, apply pressure with your thumb. Then repeat the whole procedure on your left foot.

CONVENTIONAL TREATMENT

Treatment for foot pain depends on the cause. For foot pain caused by arthritis, treatment usually combines medication, exercise, and, in the case of severe flare-ups, bed rest. Extremely painful or deformed joints may require surgery.

For bone spurs, over-the-counter or prescription anti-inflammatory painkillers are usually recommended. Foam shoe inserts can relieve pressure and pain. Surgery may be required to remove severe spurs.

Over-the-counter or prescription anti-inflammatory pain medication is typically recommended for bunions. Orthotics—specially made shoe inserts—can relieve pressure on the bunion. Surgery is sometimes recom-

mended but does not necessarily provide permanent relief.

Gout usually calls for nonsteroidal anti-inflammatories.

People with plantar fasciitis often require special arch supports, though sometimes physical therapy might be recommended.

TOUCH THERAPY
Chiropractic and Osteopathic Medicine

Chiropractic manipulation of the joints and soft tissue may ease pain and increase mobility for people with arthritis. Osteopathic physicians also can prescribe medication if necessary. For bone spurs, joint and soft-tissue manipulation alleviate the wear and tear that leads to bone spurs. Spinal adjustments alleviate structural imbalances, which can lead to bunions.

Craniosacral Therapy

Practitioners say that craniosacral therapy can alleviate chronic pain, including that from arthritis.

Massage

Massage therapy holds promise for bone spurs and plantar fasciitis: Deep-tissue massage can reduce restrictions in the fascia, which can create irritation that leads to bone spurs. Massage can also reduce discomfort associated with general foot fatigue.

Myofascial Release

Myofascial release can alleviate restrictions in connective tissue that pull muscles and bones out of place, causing wear and tear and leading to bone spurs and osteoarthritis.

Physical Therapy

Various techniques of physical therapy can bring relief from pain and restore more movement, especially for osteoarthritis. One of the modalities a physical therapist may use for arthritis pain is hydrotherapy, or treatment with water.

Reflexology

Reflexology can be especially helpful for instances of foot pain due to gout. Practitioners say that this therapy can break up deposits of uric acid that accumulate in the feet and cause pain.

Structural and Functional Techniques

Ida Rolf created her technique of Structural Integration largely because she sought relief from her own arthritis. Rolfing has helped many osteoarthritis sufferers in particular, by alleviating structural abnormalities that strain muscles, tendons, and joints. Rolfing and Hellerwork involve deep-tissue massage, which can alleviate restrictions that lead to bone spurs and bunions, too. Movement re-education also teaches patients new patterns of movement to reduce the physical stress that can lead to foot problems.

Acupressure for Pain

No matter what the source of your foot pain, pressing Gall Bladder 20 may help alleviate it. This is an anti-inflammatory point that eases pain all over the body. It is located at the back of the neck in line with the first thoracic vertebrae, two finger widths on either side of the spine.

HEADACHES

Headaches are often the result of tension in the meninges (the outer linings of the brain) and in the muscles and blood vessels of the scalp and neck. Headaches can vary in severity and scope. The pain may be mild or severe, and can be throbbing or sharp. The pain may be in only one part of the head, such as the forehead or back of the neck, or it may be felt all over.

There are several main types of headaches:

* Tension headaches typically are caused by stress or poor posture. They result when tense facial, scalp, and neck muscles press on blood vessels in the scalp, causing a dull, throbbing pain. Lack of blood flow to tissues or tension in the muscles themselves can be the source of the pain. Tension headaches may last only a day or two, or they can become chronic and recur for weeks at a time.

* Vascular headaches involve blood vessels. Migraines are the most severe type of vascular headache. They cause intense, debilitating pain and can be accompanied by visual and aural disturbances, nausea, shakiness, and vomiting. During a migraine, the patient may be extremely sensitive to environmental stimuli, including light, sound, and smell. Migraines can last a few hours or several days. More women than men experience migraines. Many women experience migraines as part of their menstrual cycle; pregnant women usually experience fewer or milder attacks. Cluster headaches also are vascular and tend to affect men more than women. They usually occur at night when a person is asleep. They involve intense, sharp pain behind one eye and can occur every day for weeks at a time.

* Sinus headaches are the result of swelling or infection in the mucous membranes of the sinuses or from congestion in the sinuses. They tend to involve pain and pressure in the upper part of the head, across the forehead and nose and behind the eyes.

Headaches can have many causes. Tension headaches are typically the result of emotional stress, but may also be caused by physical stress, such as bad posture, eyestrain, or a noisy environment.

The cause of migraines can be hard to pin down, but triggers include:

* food sensitivities
* hormonal fluctuations
* stress
* erratic sleep habits
* cigarette smoke
* altitude

Cluster headaches do not have a clear cause, though they are known to be more common in smokers.

CONVENTIONAL TREATMENT

The standard therapy for headaches is medication. Analgesics, including aspirin and acetaminophen, generally are recommended for tension headaches. Sinus headaches can be alleviated with decongestants and, if necessary, antibiotics to treat an infectious cause of the inflammation, if any.

A wide variety of medications are used to treat migraines:

* over-the-counter analgesics
* prescription painkillers
* medications that regulate blood-vessel constriction, such as beta-blockers
* antidepressants

These drugs can have serious side effects, however, and painkillers, if used for long periods of time, can have a rebound effect, which means that they actually end up causing headaches. They also may interfere with the action of endorphins.

TOUCH THERAPY

Acupressure

Pressing on the Gall Bladder 20 points can help alleviate a tension headache. These are located in the hollows at the base of the skull, about two inches out on both sides of the spine. Another useful point is on the back of each hand in the webbing between the thumb and index finger.

Aromatherapy

Peppermint essential oil is used for all types of headaches. Scents that ease anxiety and stress may alleviate tension headaches; these include:

* lavender
* marjoram
* lemon
* bergamot
* sandalwood

For a sinus headache, give eucalyptus a try.

Chiropractic and Osteopathic Medicine

Tight muscles in the upper back and neck can lead to tension headaches. Using manipulation and soft-tissue massage, a chiropractor or osteopathic physician can realign the spine and loosen muscles to alleviate the muscle strain that may be causing headaches.

Craniosacral Therapy

This form of extremely gentle manipulation focuses on alleviating tension in the membranes that encase the brain and spinal cord. Practitioners say it can be very effective at relieving headaches.

Massage

Massage reduces tension and restores blood flow in muscles throughout the body, including those in the head, neck, and shoulders that can cause or contribute to a headache. Massage also causes a number of physiologic responses that play a role in reducing anxiety and stress. Among the many benefits, it:

* slows heart rate
* lowers blood pressure
* improves digestion
* reduces levels of stress-related hormones

Finally, massage also triggers the release of endorphins, hormones that alleviate pain and create a sense of comfort and well-being.

Myofascial Release

Myofascial release can alleviate restrictions in connective tissue that pull muscles and bones out of place and contribute to headaches.

Reflexology

Massaging the big toe, which corresponds to the head, may help ease headaches. Hold the

HEADACHE-INDUCING FOODS

Certain foods have been linked to tension and migraine headaches, and if you're a sufferer, you might try eliminating them from your diet. In some cases, the foods affect blood vessels in the head, but in other cases their relationship to headaches isn't understood. Common dietary culprits include:

* aged cheeses
* caffeine
* chocolate
* citrus fruits
* hotdogs
* nuts
* red wine

big toe with the thumb and index finger of one hand. With the other hand, using the thumb as a support, roll the index finger across portions of the toe for about 30 seconds to 2 minutes; repeat on other toe. Massaging the zones connected to the head, neck, and shoulders may also be beneficial.

Therapeutic Touch

Research has shown that Therapeutic Touch prompts the relaxation response, a physiologic state in which heart and breathing rates drop, brainwave activity slows, and muscles become less tense. Levels of various body chemicals associated with stress also decline. This may be beneficial for headaches caused by stress.

Shiatsu

Shiatsu can release tension in muscles throughout the body, including the head, neck, and shoulders. One study found that shiatsu alleviated migraines in more than half the subjects.

Structural and Functional Techniques

Rolfing and Hellerwork involve deep-tissue and joint manipulations, which help to realign the body and decrease the structural imbalances that cause headaches. These, as well as the other movement re-education therapies, also teach patients new patterns of movement that can improve posture, which may alleviate headaches.

HYPERTENSION

Everyone's blood pressure occasionally goes up in reaction to physical activity and stress. A person suffers from hypertension when his blood pressure remains high even at rest. Hypertension is extremely common in developed nations, affecting about 40 million Americans. It is the primary cause of stroke and also plays a major role in heart disease.

Blood pressure is described by two numbers, systolic pressure and diastolic pressure. Systolic pressure is the first number and refers to the peak force of blood as it is pumped by the heart. Diastolic pressure is the second number and measures the force of blood as the heart fills between beats. Normal blood pressure for an adult is 120/80. Pressure of 140/90 is considered high if it is measured at this level on two occasions.

In the vast majority of hypertension cases, the cause cannot be determined. This is known as essential hypertension. There are a variety of known risk factors. Essential hypertension is more likely to affect:

* people with a family history of hypertension
* men
* blacks (as compared with whites)
* people who consume high levels of sodium
* people who are overweight
* alcoholics
* people with a sedentary lifestyle

When the cause is known, it is called secondary hypertension. Causes include kidney disease, pregnancy, and birth-control pills.

Blood pressure that is too high can damage the arteries—the blood vessels that carry blood away from the heart. If not treated, hypertension can lead to:

* vision problems
* stroke
* heart attack
* congestive heart failure

CONVENTIONAL TREATMENT

Because hypertension rarely causes any symptoms, it is important to have your blood pressure checked regularly.

Unless blood pressure is extremely high, lifestyle changes will probably be recommended before medication. These include lowering salt intake, getting regular exercise, losing weight, quitting smoking, and reducing stress.

If these changes do not make a significant enough difference, medication will likely be prescribed, including:

* angiotensin converting enzyme (ACE) inhibitors, which prevent or slow the constriction of blood vessels
* vasodilator drugs, which expand the blood vessels
* calcium channel blockers, which impede the constriction of blood vessels
* diuretics, which eliminate salt and excess fluid

RELAX AND EASE THE PRESSURE

Relaxation techniques are an important lifestyle measure you can take to lower blood pressure without medication. In addition to touch therapies for relaxation, you might want to consider exploring biofeedback, breathing exercises, hypnotherapy, meditation, music therapy, tai chi, visualization, and yoga.

---

* beta-blockers, which halt certain messages from the central nervous system

TOUCH THERAPY

Hypertension is a serious condition that requires medical attention. Alternative therapies should be used as a supplement to, rather than replacement for, conventional care.

Acupressure

Pressing on the point called Pericardium 3 can help relax the body. It is located in the elbow crease, directly above the ring finger. Pressing on Spleen 6—located four finger widths above the inside anklebone—may help normalize blood pressure. (Do not use this point if you are pregnant, because it can stimulate uterine contractions.)

Aromatherapy Massage

Lemon and marjoram essential oils are reputed to help normalize blood pressure. Scents that have sedative properties may also be beneficial, including:

* lavender
* rose
* geranium
* sandalwood

Massage

Research has shown that massage induces the relaxation response. Massage also alleviates muscle tension, which can, in turn, ease emotional tension.

INSOMNIA

Insomnia is difficulty falling asleep or staying asleep. It's a common problem; about one in three American adults suffers from insomnia. Studies have shown that people with insomnia actually sleep more than they think they do; it is the quality, rather than the quantity, of their sleep that is the problem.

Insomnia falls into several different categories:

* Transient insomnia lasts only a few days.
* Short-term insomnia continues for a few weeks.
* Chronic insomnia is ongoing for an extended period of time.

There are many possible causes of insomnia, including:

* disruption in routine (often the source of transient insomnia)
* anxiety and stress (typically are the cause of short-term insomnia)
* caffeine consumption
* lack of exercise
* erratic hours
* environmental factors, such as excessive noise
* chronic pain
* sleep apnea (a breathing problem)
* restless leg syndrome
* depression
* alcohol or drug use
* schizophrenia
* menopause
* certain medications

CONVENTIONAL TREATMENT

Though prescription sleep aids are still common, doctors do not rely on them as heavily as they once did, preferring instead to address the underlying causes of insomnia first. Anxiety, depression, breathing problems, and physical ailments require treatment specific to those conditions.

Lifestyle changes may be suggested, including:

* eliminating caffeine from your diet
* getting regular exercise
* maintaining a regular sleep schedule
* developing a routine to wind down before bedtime, such as taking a warm bath or reading a good book
* making sure the bedroom is dark and quiet enough

The Healing Power of Touch

When all else fails, medication may be prescribed, including antihistamines, barbiturates, and benzodiazepine drugs. However, these medications can cause daytime drowsiness. Barbiturates, in particular, can cause dependence and after a while may no longer be effective in inducing sleep.

TOUCH THERAPY

Acupressure

A variety of points may help relieve insomnia. Among them are two that are aimed at calming the heart and mind. Heart 7 is located on the inner arms on the wrist crease, in the hollow that is in line with the little fingers. Pericardium 6 also is on the inner arms, between the tendons three finger widths above the wrist crease. To use any of these points, press the point or massage in a small circle around it with your finger for 30 to 60 seconds.

Aromatherapy Massage

Research has found that lavender oil can induce sleep. A variety of other essential oils are believed to alleviate insomnia as well:

* cedar
* melissa
* rose
* marjoram
* neroli
* sandalwood

Jin Shin Jyutsu

The philosophy of this pressure-point technique connects different emotions with each finger. Worry is the domain of the thumb, and pressing it gently until you feel yourself relax may help alleviate anxiety that is causing insomnia.

Massage

A large number of studies have found that massage eases anxiety, which is a common cause of insomnia. Research has shown positive results specifically for reducing anxiety in cancer patients, depressed children and teenagers, women with eating disorders, and fibromyalgia patients. One study found that 30 minutes of massage a day was more effective at alleviating anxiety than a relaxation video.

Massage is reported to help a great deal in some insomnia cases. It causes a number of physiologic responses that play a role in reducing anxiety. Among the many benefits, it:

* triggers the release of endorphins (hormones that create a sense of comfort and well-being)
* reduces muscle tension
* slows heart rate
* lowers blood pressure

THE BOOTZIN TECHNIQUE

Back in the 1970s, Richard Bootzin, Ph.D., then a psychology professor at Northwestern University, developed a six-step program that has helped thousands of people sleep better.

1. Ignore the clock and go to bed only when you feel sleepy.
2. Use your bed for sleeping and sex only. Do not eat, read, or do anything else in bed.
3. If you can't fall asleep after going to bed, leave the bedroom and don't return until you feel sleepy.
4. If necessary, repeat step 3 as many times as you have to.
5. To help your body establish a natural sleeping pattern, set your alarm for the same time every morning.
6. Do not take naps.

- improves digestion
- reduces levels of stress-related hormones

Reflexology

Practitioners say anxiety may be eased by working on points connected to the diaphragm and the pituitary, thyroid, and adrenal glands.

Rolfing

One study found that after five weeks of Rolfing treatment, subjects experienced a significant decrease in anxiety. The researchers theorize that Rolfing caused a release of emotional tension that had been stored in the muscles, which in turn resulted in lower scores on a psychological test of anxiety.

Therapeutic Touch

Research has shown that Therapeutic Touch prompts the relaxation response, a physiologic state in which heart and breathing rates drop, brainwave activity slows, and muscles become less tense. Levels of various body chemicals associated with anxiety and stress also decline. Practitioners say that the therapy creates a heightened sense of self-awareness and unity with the world.

KNEE PAIN

Knee pain can come from a variety of causes. Some cases are the result of structural problems that lead to wear and tear, some are caused by injury, and still others are the result of disease or infection.

Different knee problems have different symptoms associated with them:

* Bursitis is inflammation in a bursa, one of the fluid-filled sacs that cushion pressure points in the body, mainly the joints. Overuse, injury, or prolonged pressure can lead the bursa to become filled with fluid, causing pain and swelling.
* Gout is caused by high blood levels of uric acid, which forms crystals, mainly in the big toe but other joints as well, including the knees. These crystals cause inflammation, pressure, and severe pain. A number of conditions seem to be associated with gout, but it is especially common in men who are overweight, drink alcohol, and eat rich diets full of organ meats and gravy.
* Osteoarthritis is the result of wear and tear on the joints and causes swelling, pain, and stiffness.
* Rheumatoid arthritis, an autoimmune disorder in which the body attacks its own tissue, leads to swelling, pain, and warmth in the joints, as well as stiffness.

CONVENTIONAL TREATMENT

Treatment for knee pain depends on the cause. In arthritis, treatment usually combines medication, exercise, and, in the case of severe flare-ups, bed rest. Extremely painful or deformed joints may require surgery. (See also page 127.)

For bursitis, rest, ice packs, and over-the-counter anti-inflammatory pain medication often alleviate discomfort.

For gout, nonsteroidal anti-inflammatory medication and some dietary changes are usually recommended.

TOUCH THERAPY
Chiropractic Medicine

Chiropractic manipulation of the joints and soft tissue may ease pain and increase mobility in cases of knee pain due to arthritis. For bursitis-related knee pain, manipulation can decrease pressure on the inflamed bursa and restore proper alignment and range of motion, which can ward off future bouts.

Craniosacral Therapy

Practitioners say that craniosacral therapy can alleviate chronic pain, including that from arthritis.

Massage

Research shows that massage reduces muscle tension and prompts the body to release endorphins, natural chemicals that behave like morphine, decreasing pain and producing a feeling of well-being. Massage also can be helpful for the emotional aspects of chronic pain, because it reduces anxiety and induces relaxation. Although massage right on the affected area is contraindicated for bursitis, it can alleviate tension in tissues surrounding the inflamed bursa. Massage of the tissues surrounding the knee can be helpful especially in cases where there have been previous injuries.

Myofascial Release

Myofascial release can alleviate restrictions in connective tissue that pull muscles and bones out of place and may contribute to the pain and inflammation of bursitis, osteoarthritis, and tendonitis.

Physical Therapy

Various techniques of physical therapy can bring relief from pain and restore more movement, especially for osteoarthritis. One of the modalities a physical therapist may use for arthritis pain is hydrotherapy, or treatment with water.

Structural and Functional Techniques

Ida Rolf created her technique of Structural Integration largely because she sought relief from her own arthritis. Rolfing has helped many osteoarthritis sufferers in particular, by alleviating structural abnormalities that strain muscles, tendons, and joints. Movement re-education can teach patients how to change movement habits that exacerbate osteoarthritis, bursitis, and tendonitis in the knee.

Therapeutic Touch

Practitioners say Therapeutic Touch can alleviate many forms of chronic pain, and research indicates it prompts the relaxation response.

MENOPAUSAL DISCOMFORTS

Menopause is the cessation of menstruation, which usually occurs between the ages of 45 and 55. Declining levels of estrogen cause a woman's eggs to mature less often, which leads the body to produce less progesterone. This in turn causes the uterine lining to stop thickening on a regular basis, which causes menstrual periods to become irregular before stopping altogether.

Menopause may occur in a gradual process lasting many years or happen very quickly. Some women notice subtle changes starting in their 30s, which may include irregular periods, mild flushing sensations, and premenstrual mood changes. Many women will have no menopausal symptoms whatsoever, except that their periods disappear in their 50s.

The hormonal changes of menopause can cause a variety of side effects, including:

* hot flashes
* night sweats
* vaginal dryness
* thinner skin
* hair loss
* weight gain

Psychological disturbances, such as depression, anxiety, and mood swings, have been chalked up to menopause, but they may be caused not so much by hormonal changes but as a side effect of other symptoms, such as night sweats, which disrupt sleep. Interestingly, women in cultures that view aging positively report far fewer symptoms of menopause.

CONVENTIONAL TREATMENT

If you're experiencing uncomfortable symptoms, or if you're at risk for osteoporosis or heart disease, your doctor may recommend hormone replacement therapy (HRT). Some of the proved benefits of HRT for menopausal women include protection from the bone loss of osteoporosis, protection from heart disease, improved sleep, less severe hot flashes, and less vaginal dryness.

HRT delivers estrogen— sometimes by means of pills, sometimes through skin patches or vaginal creams—to replace decreasing levels of those hormones in your body. Some doctors may add progesterone to the mix for a woman who still has a uterus because estrogen alone has been linked with an increase in the risk of uterine and breast cancer. (In fact, if you've had breast cancer, endometrial cancer, uterine fibroids, or liver disease, HRT is usually not recommended.) Other risks include headaches, bloating, and breast pain.

TOUCH THERAPY
Aromatherapy Massage

Lavender and geranium essential oils are considered to be hormone balancers and may help alleviate menopausal symptoms. Certain essential oils are believed to have estrogenic effects and may alleviate hot flashes. These include:

* clary sage
* anise
* angelica
* sage
* fennel
* coriander

Massage

Massage induces the relaxation response, which can alleviate anxiety and depression. It may improve the quality of sleep, thus decreasing the physical and emotional effects of menopause-related sleep-deprivation.

Reflexology

Massaging the zones associated with the pelvic organs may be beneficial. The uterine/prostate reflex area is found on the inside of the ankle area, midway between the back corner of the heel and the ankle bone.

MENSTRUAL PAIN

Menstrual pain—technically known as dysmenorrhea—is so common that it's considered normal for many women. In most cases, pain is caused by the body's excess production of prostaglandins, a group of fatty acids that behave like hormones. Although some prostaglandins are beneficial, others can cause pain, inflammation, and uterine contractions. To a certain extent, these contractions are necessary, because they push out menstrual blood, but excess prostaglandins can cause contractions that are so strong they become muscle spasms.

Besides excess prostaglandins, other possible causes of dysmenorrhea include:

* endometriosis, a condition in which uterine tissue grows outside the uterus—usually in the abdominal cavity—and causes painful cysts and adhesions
* uterine polyps
* uterine fibroids
* use of an intrauterine device (IUD)

CONVENTIONAL TREATMENT

Dysmenorrhea occurs most commonly in teenagers and in women who have never been pregnant. In the absence of a more serious underlying conditions, such as endometriosis or pelvic infection, treatment relies on various kinds of medication, including:

* analgesics, such as aspirin and acetaminophen
* nonsteroidal anti-inflammatory drugs, such as ibuprofen
* birth-control pills
* progesterone

There are other remedies that help to ease menstrual pain and relieve pressure. These include placing a hot-water bottle or heating pad on the abdomen, taking hot baths, and lying on the back with the knees bent. A woman who experiences dysmenorrhea before pregnancy may find that the problem is lessened after childbirth, possibly because of enlargement of the cervix or destruction of some nerve fibers in the uterus.

TOUCH THERAPY

Acupressure

Pressing on the point Liver 3 may alleviate some menstrual cramps. This point is located just below where the big toes and second toes meet, in the webbing between the bones.

Aromatherapy Massage

Certain essential oils may relieve menstrual cramps, especially when applied to the pelvic area:

* chamomile
* lavender
* marjoram
* melissa

Chiropractic Medicine

Recent research indicates that manipulating the lower back with a certain amount of force can alleviate menstrual cramps.

Massage

Research has shown that massage prompts the release of endorphins, the body's natural painkillers, which may be beneficial for dysmenorrhea. Massage focused on the lower back and the area just above the pubic bone can alleviate menstrual pain and cramping.

Dietary Help

Avoiding most animal foods—including meat, milk, cheese, and butter—may ease menstrual cramps. These foods contain arachidonic acid, which tends to increase the production of certain prostaglandins that cause pain and inflammation.

MUSCLE CRAMPS AND TENSION

Muscles are made up of special cells that have filaments that contract and relax, which creates movement. Skeletal muscles—those whose movement is voluntarily controlled by the brain—may cramp when they contract and fail to then stretch out again. Muscle cramps cause sharp, sudden pain and feel hard to the touch.

Muscle cramps can occur for a variety of reasons, including:

* an imbalance of sodium, calcium, or magnesium (possibly caused by overexertion), all of which play an important role in transmitting the nerve impulses that cause muscles to contract and relax
* fatigue of the muscle
* a sedentary lifestyle
* sitting or standing too long in one position
* overexertion that depletes the body of fluid and minerals
* thyroid problems
* smoking, which deprives muscles of oxygen
* poor circulation
* a direct blow to the muscle

CONVENTIONAL TREATMENT

Treatment of muscle cramps usually is not necessary unless they are frequent or severe. In those cases, medication may be recommended, including:

* analgesics, such as aspirin and acetaminophen
* nonsteroidal anti-inflammatory drugs, such as ibuprofen
* muscle relaxants
* quinine, to control nighttime leg cramps

Muscle cramps in the chest or arms, particularly the left arm, can be a sign of a serious heart problem and require immediate medical attention.

TOUCH THERAPY
Acupressure

Leg cramps may be relieved by pressing on the point called Bladder 57, which is located on the back of the leg in the center of the calf, halfway between the knee and the heel.

Aromatherapy Massage

Many different scents are said to ease muscle pain:

* peppermint
* eucalyptus
* lavender
* chamomile
* ginger
* rosemary

Chiropractic and Osteopathic Medicine

Spinal adjustment and soft-tissue techniques can ease muscle tension throughout the body. Spinal manipulation has been shown to be beneficial for treating low-back pain.

Reflexology

Massaging the zones that correspond to areas of muscle spasm or tightness may be beneficial. Also, treatments may improve blood circulation, leading to better distribution of oxygen and elimination of waste products, both of which can ease muscle tightness.

Shiatsu

Shiatsu massage can release muscle tension, and practitioners say it enhances the body's self-healing abilities.

Structural and Functional Techniques

Rolfing and Hellerwork emphasize deep-tissue massage, which can ease muscle tension. These therapies teach patients how to eliminate patterns of movement that cause chronic muscle tension and pain.

Sports Massage

One of the main goals of sports massage is to reduce muscle spasms and ease stiffness by removing lactic acid from the tissues. (Lactic acid is a waste product created by vigorous exercise that can cause cramping.) Direct pressure techniques typically are used. If muscle cramps are a common problem, a massage therapist can show you self-massage techniques to help ease spasms.

NAUSEA AND VOMITING

Nausea is usually a sign of stomach irritation; vomiting is the body's natural way of getting rid of the irritant. A variety of substances can cause queasiness and throwing up, such as certain foods and medicines, hormonal fluctuations, overindulgence in food or alcohol, and pathogens like bacteria and viruses. These symptoms also may be evidence of various medical conditions, including migraine headaches, head injury, shock, inner ear problems, heart attack, and cancer.

CONVENTIONAL TREATMENT

For nausea and vomiting that occur every once in a while—during the stomach "flu," for example—the best approach is to let them run their course. If these symptoms are linked to motion sickness, morning sickness, chemotherapy treatment, and other noncritical conditions, antiemetic medications may be used to block nausea and vomiting.

TOUCH THERAPY

Acupressure

Stimulating the point called Pericardium 6, or P6, has been shown to alleviate nausea and vomiting caused by chemotherapy treatment, recovery from surgery, motion sickness, and pregnancy. P6 is located on the inner arms two finger widths above the wrist crease. Also, there are elastic wristbands available—called sea bands—that apply pressure on the P6 point with plastic disks.

Aromatherapy Massage

Basil essential oil is reputed to alleviate nausea caused by radiation and chemotherapy. Other oils that ease nausea and indigestion are:

✿ chamomile ✿ dill
✿ ginger ✿ peppermint

Reflexology

Massaging various zones on the feet may be beneficial, including those connected to the:

✿ solar plexus ✿ diaphragm
✿ chest ✿ lungs
✿ esophagus ✿ stomach
✿ liver ✿ gallbladder
✿ adrenal glands

NECK PAIN

Neck pain can be caused by a variety of factors. Among them are osteoarthritis, which causes neck stiffness that doesn't abate and in fact becomes worse. Shooting neck pain that radiates toward the arms can indicate a herniated vertebral disk. (Most disk problems, however, occur in the lower back.) Whiplash involves severe pain after an event in which the neck is forcibly bent backward and forward, typically from a car crash but also from any other type of head injury. Or neck pain may quite simply be the result of poor posture, especially if you sit in front of a desk all day. Neck pain associated with stress is often caused by chronic muscle tension.

CONVENTIONAL TREATMENT

The type of treatment depends on the ailment. For osteoarthritis, standard therapy usually combines nonsteroidal anti-inflammatory drugs, exercise, and, in the case of severe flare-ups, bed rest.

A herniated disk may require simply some spinal manipulation, rest, and, if necessary, over-the-counter anti-inflammatory medications. Severe cases may require surgery.

In cases of whiplash, the patient's neck may be immobilized in a cervical collar, though it can delay healing if worn for more than a few days. Analgesic drugs can relieve pain; muscle relaxant medication may be prescribed.

TOUCH THERAPY

Acupressure

Stimulating various acupressure points may alleviate some of the pain and swelling of osteoarthritis. In particular, Gall Bladder 20 is an anti-inflammatory point that relieves pain all over the body. It is located at the back of the neck in line with the first thoracic vertebrae, two finger widths on either side of the spine.

Aromatherapy Massage

Many different scents are said to ease muscle pain, including:

* camphor
* chamomile
* eucalyptus
* ginger
* lavender
* marjoram

Chiropractic Medicine

Chiropractic treatment is particularly well suited to address neck pain. By realigning the vertebrae and joints in the spine, chiropractic manipulation can reduce neck pain in cases of herniated disk. Soft-tissue manipulation can ease muscle spasms surrounding an injured disk. In osteoarthritis, chiropractic treatments may alleviate pain for many sufferers. Misaligned spinal vertebrae and joints place abnormal stress throughout the body, which can make osteoarthritis worse. Chiropractic adjustment focuses on bringing the spine into proper alignment, which can alleviate pain and restore normal movement. Treating whiplash is, along with back pain, one of chiropractic's specialties. Once the muscle spasm of whiplash has begun to ease, a chiropractor may manipulate the spine and soft tissue to further relieve the spasms.

Craniosacral Therapy

Practitioners say they've had good results in treating whiplash, as well as the chronic pain of osteoarthritis.

Massage

Massaging the muscles in the neck can relieve tightness and help improve mobility for osteoarthritis patients. Also, massage has been shown to prompt the release of endorphins, natural chemicals that behave like morphine, killing pain and producing a sense of well-being. Massage is often used to treat the sore and damaged muscles of whiplash. It is especially useful in neck pain caused by stress and fatigue.

Myofascial Release

Myofascial release can alleviate restrictions in connective tissue that pull muscles and bones out of place, which can contribute to osteoarthritis.

Physical Therapy

Various techniques of physical therapy can bring relief from pain and restore more movement, especially for osteoarthritis. One of the modalities a physical therapist may use for arthritis pain is hydrotherapy, or treatment with water. Warm, moist heat applied in a compress can help alleviate pain and stiffness. A program of isometric exercises and swimming can help increase circulation to the affected joints and improve muscle strength without stressing the joints. Traction may be used to reduce the compression of the spine.

WHEN TO SEEK HELP

Neck pain is characteristic of meningitis, an infection of the membranes that cover the spinal cord and brain. If meningitis is caused by bacterial infection, it can be fatal in a short amount of time; viral meningitis is not quite as serious, but it can be dangerous. In any case, if you experience neck pain that is preceded by a severe headache and is accompanied by either fever, nausea, vomiting, light sensitivity, sleepiness, or confusion, seek medical attention immediately.

Structural and Functional Techniques

Rolfing and Hellerwork involve deep-tissue and joint manipulation, which realigns the body and decreases structural imbalances that cause neck pain. These as well as the other movement re-education therapies also teach patients new patterns of movement that can reduce neck pain.

Rolfing, in particular, can help osteoarthritis sufferers. Stretching the fascia—the connective tissue that surrounds muscles and connects them to the bones—can alleviate structural abnormalities that strain muscles, tendons, and joints and cause osteoarthritis. Realigning the body reduces wear and tear, improving movement and bringing relief from pain.

PARKINSON DISEASE

Parkinson disease is a brain disorder caused by degeneration of nerve cells in the basal ganglia—a part of the brain that is critical to producing muscle movements that are smooth and continuous. Over time, muscles become very tense, which causes tremors, stiff joints, weakness, and slow movement. Everyday tasks can eventually become very difficult. About a third of Parkinson patients eventually succumb to dementia.

CONVENTIONAL TREATMENT

Medication can help control the symptoms of Parkinson disease and improve the quality of life for a while, though it cannot halt the disease. The drug most commonly used is levodopa, better known as l-dopa. However, because l-dopa becomes less effective over time, doctors often try to hold off its use as long as possible. Antidepressants may be prescribed, because depression is common in patients coping with the disease. Physical therapy is often recommended.

TOUCH THERAPY

Parkinson disease is a serious condition that requires medical attention. Alternative treatments should be used only as an adjunct to, not a replacement for, conventional care.

Massage

Various kinds of massage, especially deep-tissue work, can help ease muscle tension and loosen stiff joints, which may help increase range of motion. Massage can also alleviate the depression and constipation that often are a side effect of Parkinson disease.

Structural and Functional Techniques

The deep-tissue massage techniques of Rolfing and Hellerwork can help ease muscle tension and loosen stiff joints, which may improve range of motion. Also, the Feldenkrais Method is known for its benefits to patients with neuromuscular disturbances and may be helpful. Feldenkrais teachers work with patients to re-educate their nervous system.

POSTSURGICAL RECOVERY

Surgery is never a pleasant prospect, but in many cases it is the best—indeed, sometimes the only—option. But even successful surgery can have unpleasant side effects, including fatigue, nausea, and headaches from the anesthesia, and pain, scarring, and stiffness and poor circulation from being immobile for an extended period of time.

CONVENTIONAL TREATMENT

Various medications may be prescribed to alleviate nausea and pain and to fight off other complications such as infection.

TOUCH THERAPY

Acupressure

Applying pressure to the gall-bladder points may ease fatigue as well as stimulate the immune system. Stimulating the point called Pericardium 6, or P6, has been shown to alleviate nausea and vomiting associated with anesthesia's after-effects. P6 is located on the inner arms two finger widths above the wrist crease. Also, there are elastic wristbands available—called sea bands—that apply continuous pressure on the P6 point with plastic disks.

Aromatherapy Massage

Essential oils reputed to ease nausea and indigestion include the following:

* chamomile
* ginger
* dill
* peppermint

Scents that may ease headaches include:

* lavender
* marjoram
* lemon
* Roman chamomile
* bergamot
* sandalwood
* peppermint

Scents that may help ease postsurgical pain include:

* camphor
* eucalyptus
* lavender
* peppermint
* thyme
* chamomile
* ginger
* marjoram
* rosemary

Craniosacral Therapy

Practitioners say that craniosacral therapy can alleviate headaches and musculoskeletal pain associated with long recovery times.

Massage

Massage can be helpful in alleviating many postsurgical effects. Research shows that massage reduces muscle tension and prompts the body to release endorphins, natural chemicals that behave like morphine, decreasing pain and producing a feeling of well-being. It stimulates circulation, improves localized blood flow, and can release adhesions that may lead to excessive scarring. Massage also has been found to boost energy.

Reflexology

Massaging the points corresponding to the part of the body affected by the surgery is helpful. For general nausea and vomiting, massage of various zones on the feet can be employed, including those connected to the:

- solar plexus
- chest
- esophagus
- liver
- adrenal glands
- diaphragm
- lungs
- stomach
- gallbladder

Therapeutic Touch

One study found that Therapeutic Touch accelerated wound healing. It also can reduce post-surgical pain.

Alleviating Anxiety

The period leading up to a surgical procedure can be an extremely anxious time as a patient wonders whether he's choosing the best option and whether the surgery will be successful. Touch therapy can be extremely beneficial in reducing pre-surgery jitters:

- A variety of essential oils are reputed to reduce anxiety and can be used in an aromatherapy massage. Among the most effective oils are lavender, bergamot, marjoram, sandalwood, lemon, and Roman chamomile.
- A large number of studies has found that massage eases anxiety.
- Reflexology practitioners say anxiety may be eased by working on points connected to the diaphragm and the pituitary, thyroid, and adrenal glands.
- Research has shown that Therapeutic Touch prompts the relaxation response and may help make patients more at ease before surgery.

PREGNANCY DISCOMFORTS

Though it often can be a time of great joy, pregnancy also can be a very uncomfortable experience. Hormonal changes and an expanding uterus can cause a variety of symptoms, including morning sickness, headaches, insomnia, back pain, constipation, sciatica, and fatigue.

CONVENTIONAL TREATMENT

Because of the possibility of damage to the developing fetus, very few medications are recommended to treat pregnancy discomforts. Instead, doctors recommend adopting various habits to ward off symptoms:

* For morning sickness and stomach upset, try eating several small meals throughout the day. Eating crackers before getting out of bed may ease morning sickness.
* To prevent constipation, eat ample amounts of fiber and drink at least 8 glasses of water a day.
* To beat fatigue, nap throughout the day if possible. Exercise also boosts energy.

TOUCH THERAPY

Acupressure

Check with a practitioner before using acupressure on yourself. Pressing certain points can cause uterine con-

tractions and induce miscarriage or premature labor.

For back pain, fatigue, and sciatica, try pressing Bladder 23 and Bladder 47. Bladder 23 is located on the back, level with the navel, about an inch away from the spine, on both sides. Bladder 47 is found level with Bladder 23, about an inch farther away from the spine.

Research on pregnant women found that pressing on the point called Pericardium 6, or P6, four times a day for 10 minutes helped alleviate the nausea of morning sickness. P6 is located on the inner arms two finger widths above the wrist crease. Also, there are elastic wristbands available—called sea bands—that apply pressure on P6 with plastic disks.

Aromatherapy Massage

Pregnant women should always check with a qualified health-care practitioner before using essential oils. The essential oils of clary sage and lavender can help alleviate insomnia. Ginger and peppermint essential oils can ease stomach upset.

Chiropractic and Osteopathic Medicine

For back pain and sciatica, manipulation and soft-tissue techniques can correct spinal misalignment, reduce pressure on the sciatic nerve, and relieve pain and inflammation.

Craniosacral Therapy

For back pain, headaches, and sciatica, craniosacral therapy may be especially useful in later stages of pregnancy, when chiropractic or osteopathic manipulation is not possible.

Reflexology

Massaging the big toe, which corresponds to the head, may help ease some headaches. Massaging the zones that are connected to the head, neck, and shoulders may also be beneficial. Research indicates that reflexology may also provide relief from sciatica. Try massaging the zones associated with the sciatic nerve and the hips; these zones are located on the outer ankle between the ankle bone and the Achilles tendon.

Massage

Massage can be very beneficial for the relief of the strain of pregnancy. Many massage techniques must be modified for pregnant women, so be sure to work with a massage therapist who has specific training and experience with pregnant women.

USE NATURAL CAUTION

Natural remedies like aromatherapy can be very helpful in alleviating many of the discomforts of pregnancy without the harmful side effects of drugs. Just because something is natural, however, doesn't necessarily mean it's risk free. Inhaling certain essential oils and pressing specific acupressure points, for example, can cause uterine contractions that may lead to miscarriage. Herbal medicine is another natural therapy to use very cautiously during pregnancy. Goldenseal, for instance, which is popular for fighting bacterial infections, is reported to cause uterine contractions in high doses. Before using any therapy, whether conventional or natural, you'd be wise to first check with a knowledgeable health-care practitioner.

PREMATURE BIRTH

About 10 percent of babies born in the United States are premature, delivered before 37 weeks' gestation. (Pregnancy usually lasts 40 weeks.) Premature infants tend to be very small, typically less than five-and-a-half pounds. Despite many technologic advances, many premature newborns are at very high risk of impairment and death.

CONVENTIONAL TREATMENT

Because their lungs, gastrointestinal systems, and various reflexes and body functions are underdeveloped, premature infants usually have numerous health problems and require intensive care for several weeks, or until they've reached about five pounds in weight.

Consuming enough calories is especially problematic for preemies, because their stomach capacity is so small and their sucking and swallowing reflexes are immature; many low-birth-weight babies must be fed intravenously. Babies weighing less than 3.3 pounds require fortification because breast milk doesn't provide enough calcium or protein to meet their needs.

All babies have unstable temperature regulating mechanisms—that's why they wear little knit hats for several days after birth—but low-birth-weight babies have even more difficulty. Because they have an exceptionally large body surface area in relation to their body mass, they lose heat very quickly. Keeping them warm, usually in an incubator, is key to their survival.

TOUCH THERAPY
Massage

Studies show that massage can help premature infants gain weight more rapidly. In one study, a group of premature infants, or "preemies," received three 15-minute massages per day, while another group of preemies did not receive any massage. Even though both groups had the same calorie intake, the massaged babies gained 47 percent more weight than the other babies. Massage stimulated the infants' brains to release more insulin, which helped the babies' bodies use their food more efficiently.

Massage also calms a baby's central nervous system, lowering stress hormones and putting her in a general state of relaxation. Babies who receive massage, including preemies, sleep more deeply and are more alert and responsive while awake. They also tend to experience fewer episodes of apnea, or cessation of breathing, which can cause sudden infant death syndrome (SIDS).

Craniosacral Therapy

Craniosacral therapy can help to counteract any stress sustained on the skull during birth. The malleable quality of the infant skull makes it very responsive to this technique.

PREMENSTRUAL SYNDROME

Better known as PMS, premenstrual syndrome is a constellation of symptoms that occur anywhere from 2 to 14 days before the menstrual period. Given that some medical experts don't believe PMS even exists, it's not surprising that the causes are not well established. Possible explanations include hormonal imbalances and dietary deficiencies.

It's estimated that 90 percent of women will at some point experience PMS symptoms, including:

* irritability
* depression
* fatigue
* breast tenderness
* bloating
* headache
* backache

CONVENTIONAL TREATMENT

The therapy used depends on symptoms:

* Relaxation techniques curb tension.
* Diuretics eliminate excess fluid.
* Dietary changes can correct nutrient deficiencies.

TOUCH THERAPY

Aromatherapy Massage

Essential oils may be beneficial in alleviating various symptoms of PMS. For depression, helpful oils include clary sage, neroli, jasmine, and ylang-ylang. For water retention, carrot seed, grapefruit, and juniper may be useful. For headache, try lavender or marjoram.

Massage

Massage has been shown to induce the relaxation response, which may ease tension, irritability, and depression. Massage of the lower abdominal area between the pubic bone and the navel may be helpful.

Reflexology

A small study found that reflexology eased PMS symptoms. The researchers for the study speculate that reflexology may have reduced certain biochemical reactions to stress, which exacerbates PMS symptoms.

Therapeutic Touch

Practitioners contend that Therapeutic Touch can alleviate many PMS symptoms.

SCIATICA

Sciatica is pain radiating from the sciatic nerve, which runs from the lower lumbar spine down both legs to the feet—the longest nerve in the body. Occasionally, pain will involve the entire nerve, but it more typically is localized in one area. Severe cases may involve muscle weakness or numbness in the leg or foot.

The primary cause of sciatica is disk prolapse, in which the inner core of a vertebral disk bulges out and presses on the sciatic nerve at its root. Other causes of sciatica include:

* poor posture
* a mattress that is too soft
* sports injury
* pressure on the nerve by a contracted muscle (particularly the piriform muscle deep in the buttocks area)
* pregnancy
* osteoarthritis
* in rare cases, a tumor, abscess, or blood clot

CONVENTIONAL TREATMENT

Because the reason for sciatica often is not known, the main approach is simply to relieve the pain with medication, such as:

* analgesics, such as aspirin and acetaminophen
* nonsteroidal anti-inflammatory drugs, such as ibuprofen

* prescription painkillers
* corticosteroids

TOUCH THERAPY

Acupressure

Pressing on the Bladder 23 point may help relieve sciatica. It is located on the back, level with the navel, about an inch away from the spine, on both sides.

Chiropractic and Osteopathic Medicine

Manipulation and soft-tissue techniques can reduce pressure on the sciatic nerve and relieve pain and inflammation.

Massage

Various types of massage can reduce muscle tension, easing pain and inflammation. Massage of the piriform muscle may bring relief.

Myofascial Release

Myofascial release can alleviate restrictions in connective tissue that pull muscles and bones out of place, which can contribute to pain in the sciatic nerve.

Physical Therapy

Physical therapists are qualified to diagnose and treat problems related to physical function, including sciatica. Physical therapists have a wide variety of modalities at their disposal, including:

* relaxation exercises
* biofeedback
* electrical stimulation
* hydrotherapy
* heat
* ultrasound
* ice therapy
* manipulation
* therapeutic massage

Physical therapy also is beneficial for developing a preventive program of exercise and movement strategies.

Reflexology

Research indicates that reflexology may provide relief from sciatica. Try massaging the zones associated with the sciatic nerve and the hips.

Shiatsu

The deep-tissue techniques of shiatsu may ease restrictions that can cause sciatic pain. Sciatica is often related to back pain; one study found that two weekly shiatsu massages provided significant relief of chronic back pain for the majority of subjects, many of whom had not responded to mainstream treatment or even acupuncture.

Structural and Functional Techniques

Rolfing and Hellerwork involve deep-tissue and joint manipulation, which realigns the body and decreases structural imbalances that may cause sciatica. These as well as the other movement re-education therapies also teach patients new patterns of movement that can reduce sciatic pain.

SHOULDER PAIN

Shoulder pain can come from a variety of causes.
Some cases are the result of structural problems that
lead to wear and tear, some are caused by injury,
and still others are the result of disease or infection.

Different shoulder problems have different symptoms associated with them. Here are some common shoulder problems:

* Bursitis is inflammation in a bursa, one of the fluid-filled sacs that cushion pressure points in the body, mainly the joints. Overuse, injury, or prolonged pressure can result in the bursa becoming filled with fluid, causing pain and swelling.
* Gout is caused by high blood levels of uric acid, which forms crystals, mainly in the big toe but in other joints as well, sometimes the shoulders. These crystals cause inflammation, pressure, and severe pain. A number of conditions seem to be associated with gout, but it is especially common in men who are overweight, drink alcohol, and eat rich diets full of organ meats and gravy.
* Osteoarthritis is the result of wear and tear on the joints and causes pain and stiffness.
* Rheumatoid arthritis, an autoimmune disorder in which the body attacks its own tissue, leads to swelling, pain, and warmth in the joints, as well as stiffness and limited range of motion.
* Tendinitis is an inflammation of the tendons, typically as a result of repetitive motion.

CONVENTIONAL TREATMENT

Treatment for shoulder pain depends on the cause. For arthritis, treatment usually combines medication, exercise, and, in the case of severe flare-ups, bed rest. Extremely painful or deformed joints may require surgery.

Rest, ice packs, and over-the-counter anti-inflammatory pain medication often alleviate bursitis and gout. Tendinitis may require icing, and nonsteroidal anti-inflammatory drugs typically are used to ease the pain of tendinitis.

TOUCH THERAPY

Chiropractic Medicine

Chiropractic manipulation of the joints and soft tissue may ease pain and increase mobility in arthritis cases. In bursitis, manipulation can decrease pressure on the inflamed bursa and restore proper alignment and range of motion.

Craniosacral Therapy

Practitioners say that craniosacral therapy can alleviate chronic pain, including that from arthritis.

Massage

In arthritis, research shows that massage reduces muscle tension and prompts the body to release endorphins, natural chemicals that behave like morphine, decreasing pain and producing a feeling of well-being. Massage also can be helpful for the emotional aspects of chronic pain, because it reduces anxiety and induces relaxation. In bursitis, massage is contraindicated right on the affected area, but it can alleviate tension in tissues surrounding the inflamed bursa. It is effective, however, for tendinitis such as rotator-cuff tendinitis.

Myofascial Release

Myofascial release can alleviate restrictions in connective tissue that pull muscles and bones out of place—all contributing factors in bursitis, osteoarthritis, and tendinitis.

Osteopathic Medicine

Osteopathic manipulation of the joints and soft tissue may ease pain and increase mobility in arthritis. Osteopathic physicians also can prescribe medication if necessary.

Physical Therapy

Various techniques of physical therapy can bring relief from pain and restore more movement, especially for osteoarthritis. One of the modalities a physical therapist may use for arthritis pain is hydrotherapy, or treatment with water.

Structural and Functional Techniques

Ida Rolf created her technique of Structural Integration largely because she sought relief from her own arthritis. Rolfing has helped many osteoarthritis sufferers in particular, by alleviating structural abnormalities that strain muscles, tendons, and joints, including the shoulder. Movement re-education can teach patients how to change movement habits that exacerbate osteoarthritis, bursitis, and tendinitis.

SINUSITIS

Sinusitis is an inflammation of the membrane that lines the sinuses. Most of the time, sinusitis is caused by a bacterial infection that occurs as a side effect of a viral infection, but sometimes it is the result of a tooth abscess or facial injury. Sinusitis can cause severe pain in the face, and it often is accompanied by fever and congestion.

CONVENTIONAL TREATMENT

Antibiotics are prescribed to eliminate the infection. A decongestant (spray or oral) medication may be recommended to alleviate inflammation and improve drainage of the sinuses. If the sinuses are infected, antibiotics may be necessary.

TOUCH THERAPY

Acupressure

To alleviate pain and swelling, press Large Intestine 20. It is located on both sides of the bottom of the nose, next to the outer edge of the nostrils.

Aromatherapy Massage

Essential oils of eucalyptus, pine, and thyme can help eliminate congestion.

Massage

Manual lymph drainage improves circulation of the lymph, a fluid that carries white blood cells and is important to immune function. It also reduces chronic inflammation.

ANCIENT YOGI SECRET

Rinsing the sinuses each day can help prevent sinusitis. This is the traditional practice in yoga, which emphasizes the importance of clear, deep breathing. The easiest way to do a nasal wash is with a neti pot, which is available at many natural food stores. Mix about half a teaspoon of non-iodized salt with a potful of warm water. Lean your head over a basin or sink, then rotate your head to the right. Gently insert the spout of the neti pot into the right nostril, then raise the pot until water flows out the left nostril. Repeat, this time rotating the head to the left and inserting the spout in the left nostril.

SPORTS INJURIES

Although injury is extremely common in athletics, what are typically thought of as sports injuries can occur during other activities as well. For instance, although tennis elbow does affect a large number of tennis players, the majority of sufferers incur the injury during activities involving repetitive motion, such as carpentry.

Among the range of injuries common during sports activities are:

* back and neck injuries, especially herniated disks, which involve protrusion of one or more vertebral disks in the spine
* bone fractures
* charley horse, a painful knot caused by fluid accumulating around torn muscle fibers
* head injuries such as concussion, in which a blow to the head or neck interferes with electrical activity in the brain and causes a brief period of unconsciousness
* joint dislocation, which involves displacement of the bones in the joint so that they're no longer in contact with one another. It also usually includes tearing of the ligaments in the joint
* plantar fasciitis, an inflammation of the connective tissue in the foot that tends to occur in people who walk or run a lot
* shin splints, or pain in the front or sides of the lower leg, typically caused by inflammation of a muscle or tendon there
* sprains, or the tearing or stretching of a ligament, the tough bands of tissue that hold bones together
* strains, or the tearing or stretching of a muscle when it's suddenly pulled too far
* tendinitis, an inflammation of the tendons, which are the flexible cords that join muscles to each other and to bones
* muscle spasm, an intense contraction of muscle fibers causing pain and lack of movement

CONVENTIONAL TREATMENT

The standard treatment approach depends on the injury.

The Healing Power of Touch

- Bone fractures must be treated by a professional to realign and immobilize them for several weeks while they heal.

- Charley horses, plantar fasciitis, shin splints, minor sprains and strains, and tendinitis typically are treated with rest, ice packs, and anti-inflammatory medications. Arch supports may help alleviate plantar fasciitis, though sometimes physical therapy might be recommended.

- Head injuries should always be treated by a medical professional. Concussions require at least 24 hours of rest and observation; symptoms that do not abate may indicate internal bleeding, which requires surgery.

- Care for herniated disks usually involves nonsteroidal anti-inflammatory medications, moderately restricted activity for a few days, and spinal manipulation and/or physical therapy.

- Joint dislocation requires professional treatment to manipulate the joint back into place, often with the use of a general anesthetic. Then the joint is immobilized with a splint or cast for several weeks while it heals.

TOUCH THERAPY
Applied Kinesiology

Applied kinesiologists can help alleviate structural imbalances that may lead to tendinitis.

Aromatherapy Massage

Lavender essential oil is said to alleviate inflammation in soft tissue, which may be helpful. However, do not massage directly on an inflammation, focusing instead on the surrounding area.

Many different scents are said to ease muscle pain, including:

- camphor
- eucalyptus
- lavender
- peppermint
- thyme
- chamomile
- ginger
- marjoram
- rosemary

Chiropractic Medicine

Treating back pain is chiropractic's specialty. Chiropractors treat back pain by manipulating the vertebrae and joints in the spine, restoring them to their proper positions. Numerous studies, including a report from the U.S. government, have found spinal manipulation to be the safest, most effective therapy for acute back pain. Research also shows that compared to back-pain patients who use standard medical care, chiropractic patients experience greater improvement, lower health care costs, and fewer lost work days, and are more satisfied with their care.

Craniosacral Therapy

Practitioners say that craniosacral therapy can alleviate chronic pain, including back pain. An advanced craniosacral technique called unwinding focuses on releasing specific trauma from the body by recreating the position of the body when the trauma occurred, which may be helpful if back pain is the result of injury.

Massage

Sports massage is a specialty area in which massage therapists may become certified through the American Massage Therapy Association. Sports massage can enhance warm-up before exercise or competition and prevent injury, improve performance, and reduce muscle spasms and ease stiffness after an event by removing lactic acid from the tissues. (Lactic acid is a waste product created by vigorous exercise that can cause cramping.) In cases of injury—including charley horses, shin splints, sprains, strains, and tendinitis—sports massage can improve circulation in the affected area, aid removal of waste products, alleviate swelling, and speed recovery. Sports massage can also be used in training to prevent injury, speed recovery, and reduce the incidence of soreness.

Myofascial Release

Myofascial release can alleviate restrictions in connective tissue that pull muscles and bones out of place, which can contribute to tendinitis.

Osteopathic Medicine

Studies have shown that osteopathic manipulation can decrease recovery time in cases of back pain. Spinal manipulation, including that performed by osteopathic physicians, is among the primary treatment recommended for back pain by the U.S. government. Because osteopaths are qualified to prescribe, medication may also be recommended.

Physical Therapy

Physical therapists can treat many sports injuries, including charley horses, shin splints, sprains, strains, and tendinitis. Physical therapists have a wide variety of modalities at their disposal, including:

* electrical stimulation
* hydrotherapy   * traction
* heat   * ultrasound
* ice therapy   * laser therapy

HOLD OFF ON HEAT

When a sports injury occurs, you may be inclined to apply heat to the area because it feels soothing. But heat can increase swelling if applied too soon. For the first 24 hours after the onset of pain, apply ice to the painful area, to reduce inflammation. After a day or two, use moist heat, such as a wet washcloth, to stimulate blood circulation to the area, which increases the removal of waste products and speeds healing.

The goal is to alleviate pain, inflammation, and muscle tension and prevent recurrence. Physical therapy can also be beneficial in restoring full range of movement after injuries such as bone fractures and joint dislocation.

Structural and Functional Techniques

With their emphasis on training patients to move in ways that reduce physical strain, the various types of movement re-education can help prevent sports injuries and improve athletic performance.

Trigger Point Therapy

Various trigger point techniques can help reduce pain that may radiate from areas of inflammation in the case of charley horses, shin splints, sprains, strains, and tendinitis.

SPRAINS AND STRAINS

Sprains and strains are two of the most common injuries around. Sprains involve the tearing or stretching of a ligament, the tough bands of tissue that hold bones together at the joints. Strains occur when muscles tear or stretch because they're suddenly pulled too far. Sprains and strains are among the typical sports injuries, but they can also happen from a fall or improperly lifting a heavy object. Also, people who are overweight or out of shape are more prone to these injuries.

CONVENTIONAL TREATMENT

It's important that sprains and strains be allowed to heal properly. If the injured area remains out of alignment or in a weakened state, a person is prone to re-injury. If the injury isn't severe, the usual treatment is nonsteroidal anti-inflammatory medications combined with rest and ice packs.

TOUCH THERAPY
Applied Kinesiology

Applied kinesiologists can help alleviate structural imbalances that may remain after a sprain or strain.

Aromatherapy Massage

Lavender essential oil is said to alleviate inflammation in soft tissue, which may be helpful. However, do not massage directly on an inflammation; focus instead on the surrounding area.

Many different scents are said to ease muscle pain, including:

- camphor
- eucalyptus
- lavender
- peppermint
- thyme
- chamomile
- ginger
- marjoram
- rosemary

Chiropractic Medicine

Chiropractic is especially effective for treating strain in the back muscles, a common cause of back pain. Chiropractors treat back pain by manipulating the vertebrae and joints in the spine, restoring them to their proper positions. Numerous studies, including a report from the U.S. government, have found spinal manipulation to be the safest, most effective therapy for acute back pain.

Massage

In cases of sprain or strain, massage can improve circulation in the affected area, aid removal of waste products, alleviate swelling, speed recovery, and improve the tissue-healing process.

Physical Therapy

Heat treatment, ultrasound, and transcutaneous electrical nerve stimulation (TENS) from a physical therapist may help alleviate pain, inflammation, and muscle tension and reduce healing time.

Structural and Functional Techniques

Structural and functional techniques can be helpful in correcting structural misalignments caused by sprains and strains, which may be beneficial in preventing recurrence. With their emphasis on training patients to move in ways that reduce physical strain, these therapies also can help prevent sprains and strains in the first place.

Trigger Point Therapy

Trigger point techniques can help reduce pain that may radiate from areas of inflammation in the case of sprains and strains.

The RICE Remedy

The treatment known as RICE is a common approach to sprains and strains. RICE stands for rest, ice, compression, and elevation. That is:

* Avoid using the injured area.
* Apply ice packs for the first two days after injury, to ease swelling.
* Wrap the injury with an elastic pressure bandage to reduce swelling.
* Elevate the injury to help remove waste products and fluid.

When a sprain or strain happens, you may be inclined to apply heat to the area because it feels soothing. But heat can increase swelling if applied too soon. For the first 24 to 48 hours after injury, apply only ice to the painful area, to reduce inflammation. After a day or two, use moist heat, such as a wet washcloth or a hot-water bottle wrapped in a moist towel, to stimulate blood circulation to the area, which increases the removal of waste products and speeds healing.

STRESS

Stress can mean any number of things, but generally negative stress is any circumstance or situation that interferes with a person's mental health and well-being. Whether or not something is a stressor depends largely on an individual's reaction to it. An argument with a coworker may leave one person relatively unruffled, whereas someone else might feel totally overwhelmed and unable to cope with the situation. Stress takes a huge toll: Experts estimate that as much as 80 percent of illness is stress related.

When faced with a stressful situation, the body ups its production of hormones such as cortisol and epinephrine. This, in turn, causes a rise in heart rate and blood pressure, tension in the muscles, and dilation of the pupils. This reaction—known as the fight-or-flight response—can be beneficial when it helps a person fight off or avoid danger. Stress is thought to be a common cause of everyday aches and pains. Continued anxiety and stress reactions can weaken the immune system and contribute to a wide range of health problems, including:

* asthma
* back pain
* cancer
* chronic fatigue syndrome
* depression
* gastrointestinal problems
* headaches
* heart disease
* high blood pressure
* insomnia

CONVENTIONAL TREATMENT

Lifestyle factors are an important aspect of reducing stress. Doctors are likely to recommend using exercise and relaxation techniques and avoiding caffeine, alcohol, and nicotine. Talking about your feelings with a therapist can help you change your perceptions of stressful events, particularly those that cannot be avoided. A therapist or counselor may be able to help you manage your time, help you deal with stress on the job, or help you improve your family relationships. In some cases, anti-

The Healing Power of Touch

anxiety or antidepressant medications may be prescribed.

TOUCH THERAPY
Aromatherapy Massage

Alleviating stress is one of aromatherapy's specialties. A variety of scents are reputed to ease stress and induce relaxation, including:

- bergamot
- chamomile
- clary sage
- lavender
- lemon
- marjoram
- sandalwood
- neroli
- peppermint
- rose

Massage

A large number of studies have found that massage eases anxiety and stress. Research has shown positive results specifically for reducing anxiety in cancer patients, depressed children and teenagers, women with eating disorders, and fibromyalgia patients. One study found that 30 minutes of massage a day was more effective at alleviating anxiety than a relaxation video.

One of the best remedies for stress is relaxation. Because massage can have a strong relaxation effect, it can be extremely helpful. Massage causes a number of physiologic responses that play a role in promoting relaxation. Among its many benefits, massage:

- triggers the release of endorphins, hormones that create a sense of well-being
- reduces muscle tension
- slows heart rate
- lowers blood pressure
- improves digestion
- reduces levels of stress-related hormones

Reflexology

Practitioners say that a reflexology session that works all the zones of the feet can help alleviate stress.

BEAT STRESS WITH TAI CHI

Physical exercise is an excellent way to combat stress because it prompts the release of endorphins, the body's natural painkillers, which produce a sense of comfort and well-being. One activity to consider exploring is tai chi. This ancient Chinese practice uses breathing techniques and slow, graceful movements to enhance the flow of qi, the body's vital life energy. One study found that when exposed to stressful situations, subjects who practiced tai chi produced lower levels of stress hormones and showed less mood disturbance than subjects who did not.

Rolfing

One study found that after 5 weeks of Rolfing treatment, subjects experienced a significant decrease in anxiety.

The researchers theorize that Rolfing caused a release of emotional tension that had been stored in the muscles, which in turn resulted in lower scores on a psychological test of anxiety.

Therapeutic Touch

Research has shown that Therapeutic Touch, like massage, prompts the relaxation response. Studies using hospital patients found that Therapeutic Touch was more effective than simple touch in alleviating anxiety. Practitioners say that the therapy creates a heightened sense of self-awareness and unity with the world.

STROKE

A stroke occurs when the blood supply to part of the brain is cut off by a blood clot or when a blood vessel in the brain ruptures. About a third of strokes are fatal; a third of stroke victims have some lasting impairment; and a third experience no permanent effects at all.

Among the possible effects of a stroke are:

* paralysis
* speech impairment
* mental handicap
* blurred vision
* incontinence

CONVENTIONAL TREATMENT

If you suspect you or someone else is having a stroke, seek medical attention immediately, because delayed treatment can worsen the damage. Certain medication can minimize brain damage as much as possible. Surgery may be required to stop bleeding in the brain. Once the patient enters the recovery phase, medication may be prescribed to lower blood pressure or thin the blood. Rehabilitation therapy, such as speech and physical therapies, can be quite intense for several weeks or months, to help the brain learn to compensate for areas of lost function.

TOUCH THERAPY

Stroke is a critical condition that requires medical treatment. Alternative therapies should be used only as an adjunct to, never a replacement for, conventional care.

Chiropractic and Osteopathic Medicine

Chiropractic manipulation may be helpful in reducing muscle tension, increasing range of motion, and improving the function of the nervous system.

Massage

Various types of massage can improve blood circulation and flexibility in parts of the body affected by a stroke, which helps alleviate tension and pain.

Physical Therapy

Physical therapy is an important part of a stroke recovery program. The goal is to help patients regain as much normal physical function as quickly as possible. Treatments are meant

AVOIDING A STROKE

Lifestyle factors play a large role in the risk of stroke, and there are many steps you can take to reduce your chances of suffering one:

* High blood pressure is a significant stroke risk. Reducing salt intake, as well as adopting the measures below, can help lower blood pressure.
* Keep your cholesterol levels low by watching your fat intake, particularly that of saturated fats and trans fatty acids.
* Avoid a sedentary lifestyle by exercising regularly.
* Keep your weight within healthful limits; obesity raises risk.
* Do not use stimulant drugs, such as amphetamines.
* Quit smoking.
* Avoid birth control pills, which are a risk factor.
* Stress can increase the likelihood of stroke, so find ways to relax on a regular basis.

to relieve pain, increase strength and range of motion, and prevent injury. In some cases physical therapists must help patients relearn how to perform the most basic tasks of everyday living, such as dressing or bathing.

Physical therapists have a wide variety of modalities at their disposal, including:

* joint mobilization
* relaxation exercises
* biofeedback
* electrical stimulation
* hydrotherapy
* ultrasound
* laser therapy
* manipulation
* therapeutic massage

In addition, a number of therapists are incorporating more alternative approaches, including acupressure, craniosacral therapy, the Alexander Technique, the Feldenkrais Method, and Therapeutic Touch.

Structural and Functional Techniques

The Feldenkrais Method is known for its benefits to patients with neuromuscular disturbances and may be helpful in the case of stroke. Feldenkrais teachers work with patients to re-educate their nervous system, reprogramming it to adopt new ways of moving, which can be especially helpful in cases of paralysis or impaired movement.

The Healing Power of Touch

TEMPOROMANDIBULAR JOINT DISORDER (TMD)

Temporomandibular joint disorder, better known as TMD or TMJ syndrome, affects the joint that opens and closes the mouth. When this joint, as well as the muscles and ligaments connected to it, do not function properly, a person may experience pain in the jaw, face, and even the neck and shoulders, as well as headaches. Other symptoms of TMD include clicking or popping sounds when opening or closing the mouth and pain when yawning or chewing.

TMD is typically the result of tightness or spasm in the muscles that operate the temporomandibular joint, which can be caused by clenching or grinding the teeth. An improper bite also can cause tension in these muscles. Some cases are created when the joint is displaced by injuries to the jaw, as well as the head and neck.

CONVENTIONAL TREATMENT

The goal in treating TMD is to alleviate pain, reduce muscle tension, and correct underlying structural problems. Analgesics, such as aspirin and acetaminophen, usually are recommended to reduce pain. Patients may be advised to eat only soft foods for a few days, to limit chewing. Applying heat or ice to the jaw can relieve pain, as can massaging the muscles in the jaw. If the underlying problem is teeth-grinding, the patient may be fitted with a plastic bite guard or splint to wear at night.

TOUCH THERAPY
Acupressure

Applying pressure to the Stomach 7 and Large Intestine 4 points may help ease muscle tension and pain associated with TMD. Stomach 7 is located one thumb width in front of the ears, in the hollow of the upper jaw. Large Intestine 4 is in the webbing between the thumbs and index fingers. (Do not use this point if you are pregnant, however, because it may stimulate uterine contractions.)

BIOFEEDBACK BENEFITS

If your TMD is caused by stress-induced teeth-clenching, biofeedback may be the solution. Biofeedback uses electronic equipment to monitor a person's physiological responses, then gives feedback about the responses in either visual or auditory form. For instance, one type of machine measures muscle tension, producing a sound that varies as that tension increases or decreases.

Patients are taught how to control their unconscious responses to produce desired effects on the monitoring equipment. The goal is for the patient to eventually exert this control on her own, without feedback from the equipment. In the case of TMD, biofeedback can help patients learn to relax jaw and facial muscles and reduce stress levels, which in turn reduces teeth-clenching and grinding.

Chiropractic and Osteopathic Medicine

Manipulation can ease muscle tension that is contributing to TMD. Chiropractors and osteopathic physicians also can treat the neck, shoulder, and back pain that TMD patients often suffer.

Craniosacral Therapy

By manipulating the craniosacral system, practitioners say that they can correct misalignments in the bones of the skull, which can result in TMD pain.

Massage

Massage can alleviate general stress as well as reduce specific muscle tension in the jaw muscles that contributes to TMD.

Structural and Functional Techniques

The deep-tissue massage of Rolfing has been reported to alleviate TMD pain.

TENDINITIS

Tendinitis involves inflammation of the tendons, the flexible cords that join muscles to each other and to bones. Tendinitis typically occurs because of repetitive movements that overstress the tendons, but it also can be caused by injuries or infection. Exercising without warming up properly leaves many people susceptible to tendinitis.

CONVENTIONAL TREATMENT

Standard treatment for tendinitis involves nonsteroidal anti-inflammatory medications, such as ibuprofen. Corticosteroid drugs may be injected around the tendon to reduce inflammation. Ultrasound can reduce inflammation and speed the healing process.

TOUCH THERAPY

Applied Kinesiology

Applied kinesiologists can help alleviate structural imbalances that may lead to tendinitis.

Aromatherapy Massage

Lavender essential oil is said to alleviate inflammation in soft tissue. However, do not massage directly on an inflamed tendon; focus instead on the surrounding area.

Chiropractic Medicine

Chiropractic adjustments and soft-tissue manipulation can benefit most musculoskeletal problems, including tendinitis. Manipulation can restore proper alignment and range of motion.

Massage

Friction techniques promote healing of the tendons. Massage can also alleviate tension in tissues surrounding the inflamed tendon.

Myofascial Release

Myofascial release can alleviate restrictions in connective tissue that pull muscles and bones out of place, which can contribute to tendinitis.

Physical Therapy

Physical therapy may use a variety of techniques for treating tendinitis, including:

* deep-tissue massage
* electrical stimulation
* ultrasound
* stretching

The goal is to alleviate pain, inflammation, and tension and prevent recurrence.

Osteopathic Medicine

Osteopathic adjustments and soft-tissue manipulation can benefit most musculoskeletal problems, including tendinitis. Manipulation can restore proper alignment and range of motion.

Reflexology

Massaging the zone that corresponds to the area where a tendon is inflamed may provide relief. If, for instance, you have tendonitis in your knee, you would work the area on the outer edge of the foot, just in front of the heel.

Structural and Functional Techniques

Practitioners of the Alexander Technique report success in alleviating repetitive stress injuries. With their emphasis on training patients to move in ways that reduce physical strain, it is likely that many other types of movement re-education also can help treat and prevent tendinitis from occuring.

In particular, Aston-Patterning emphasizes ergonomic training, which teaches clients how to restructure their home and work environments in order to alleviate physical strain. For instance, changing the positions of a desk chair and computer is a simple measure that may prove to be beneficial.

Trigger Point Therapy

Various trigger point techniques can help reduce pain that may radiate from inflamed tendons.

TINNITUS

Tinnitus is a ringing, hissing, or buzzing noise in the ears that comes not from the outside environment but from within the head or ear itself. The noise may be due to a variety of causes, most notably repeated exposure to loud noise but also excessive wax in the ear, infection, and certain drugs, including aspirin, various antibiotics, and quinine medicines.

CONVENTIONAL TREATMENT

If tinnitus is the result of an underlying condition, such as infection or overabundant earwax, the approach is to treat that condition. If, however, tinnitus is chronic, medication may be prescribed to try to reduce the noise. Various kinds of devices worn in the ear may also be helpful.

TOUCH THERAPY

Acupressure

Try pressing the Kidney 3 point. It is located between the Achilles tendons and the inner side of the ankle bone.

Chiropractic Medicine

Chiropractic manipulation of the neck can help improve blood flow to the area, which may be beneficial.

Massage

Though massage isn't likely to alleviate tinnitus itself, it is proven to reduce stress, which is a common side effect of having tinnitus.

Osteopathic Medicine

Osteopathic manipulation of the neck oftentimes can help improve the blood flow to the area, which may prove to be beneficial.

DEALING WITH TINNITUS

The ability to cope with tinnitus varies from person to person. Some find it practically unbearable, while others experience relatively little stress from the condition. In many cases, biofeedback and hypnotherapy can help sufferers gain control over tinnitus and feel calmer. Another technique to try is machines or audiotapes that mask tinnitus with "white noise," such as the sound of running water or waves.

Whiplash

Whiplash is an injury to the muscles, ligaments, or joints of the neck, technically known as the cervical spine. Whiplash is the result of the neck being forcibly bent backward and forward, typically from a car crash but also from other types of head injury. The damage from whiplash may include a sprain of the ligaments in the neck or dislocation of a cervical joint. Pain from whiplash tends to be delayed and is usually worse a day after the injury occurs.

Whiplash may involve other symptoms besides neck pain. Other possible symptoms include dizziness, difficulty controlling movements, and loss of bladder or bowel control. A doctor should be consulted immediately if any of these symptoms are present or if pain does not begin to resolve within a day of onset.

CONVENTIONAL TREATMENT

The patient's neck may be immobilized in a cervical collar, though it can delay healing if worn for more than a few days. Analgesic drugs and muscle relaxants may be prescribed.

TOUCH THERAPY

Chiropractic Medicine

Treating whiplash is, along with back pain, one of chiropractic's specialties. Once the muscle spasm of whiplash has begun to ease, a chiropractor may manipulate the spine and soft tissue to further relieve the spasms and decrease pain.

Craniosacral Therapy

Practitioners say they've had good results in treating whiplash by addressing the affected cerebrospinal tissues.

Osteopathic Medicine

Manipulation of the spine and soft tissue can relieve muscle spasms and decrease pain.

Rolfing

Research indicates that Rolfing may be beneficial for treating whiplash.

Massage

Massage can be useful in the healing of soft tissues damaged by the trauma of whiplash.

Choosing a Practitioner

Finding the right practitioner is an important part of whether your experience is positive or negative. A therapist may be (and should be) well educated, licensed, and very experienced, but if you don't feel compatible, you're not going to be satisfied with your treatment.

INTUITION

If you don't feel comfortable with a practitioner for any reason, listen to your intuition and seek out another. As with medical doctors, a relationship with a touch therapist should be built on respect, trust, and clear communication. If a practitioner isn't willing to take the time to explain what he's doing and what your options are, feel free to find one who will.

One way to find a practitioner is by seeking referrals from friends and family members whose judgment you trust. They can tell you things that may be just as important to you as having the right credentials, for instance, what the person's office environment is like and whether she talks or is silent during the treatment.

CREDENTIALS

Having said that, though, it should also be said that credentials do matter, because they show that a person has met certain standards. Two important credentials to understand are *certification* and *licensure*. The differences between these credentials can be very confusing, especially in the case of certification, a rather murky term. To help understand the differences, let's first take a close look at each type of credential.

Certification means vouching that a practitioner has met certain specific standards. Professional certification is a voluntary process offered by some sort of private, nongovernmental organization, including many of the associations that represent different types of touch therapy. The qualifications for certification typically encompass education and written and practical exams; they may also include a certain level of experience. In order to maintain certification,

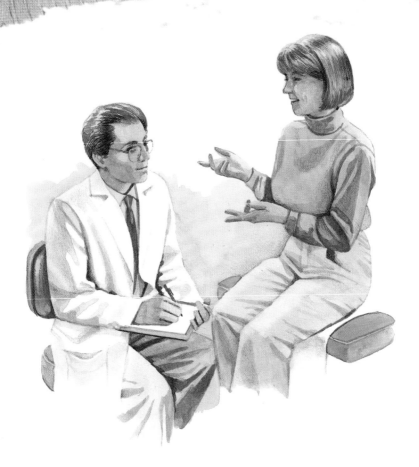

practitioners typically must meet certain continuing education requirements and then recertify within a specified period of time.

To become a certified Rolfer, a person must successfully complete the training course at the Rolf Institute, which includes more than 600 hours of lecture, observation, and hands-on experience. Practitioners must undergo advanced train-ing within five years in order to maintain their certification. In addition, they must agree to abide by a formal code of ethics and standards of practice.

Whether or not certification is meaningful depends on the credibility of the organization that does the certifying. A number of certifying bodies are, in turn, accredited by other organizations. For example, the credential Nationally Certified in Therapeutic Massage and Bodywork is awarded by the National Certification Board for Therapeutic Massage and Bodywork (NCBTMB) to individuals who meet the education and experience requirements and pass a national exam. The NCBTMB is accredited by the National Commission for Certifying Agencies, an independent agency that sets national standards for professional certification programs. Being accredited by this commission means that the NCBTMB has met rigorous standards and gives its stamp of approval enormous credibility.

Licensure is a nonvoluntary process in which the government regulates a profession. To obtain a license, a practitioner must meet certain requirements that prove he has achieved a level of competency that reasonably protects the health, safety, and welfare of patients. Licenses for healthcare professionals generally are granted at the state level; once a state has passed a licensing law for a particular occupation, it is illegal for anyone to practice or use the title of that profession in that state without a license.

Massage therapists, for example, are licensed in 25 states plus the District of Columbia; practicing massage therapy without a license is illegal in these states but not in the other 25 states that do not have licensing laws. Chiropractors, osteopathic physicians, and physical therapists are licensed in all states as well as the District of Columbia, so practicing these professions without a license anywhere in the United States is illegal. Other touch therapies, such as Rolfing, Trager, and Feldenkrais, are not licensed in any states; practitioners of these methods sometimes obtain a massage therapist license.

The difference between licensure and certification is that licensure is mandatory and certification is voluntary; one does not need to be certified to practice a particular profession. Practitioners seek out certification because it enhances their credibility by proving that they have met certain minimum standards. Certification may be required in order for a practitioner to use a certain title or copyrighted name, as in the case of Rolfers or Trager practitioners.

Another credential to look at is what sort of training a person has received. The level of training can vary enormously, depending on the profession. It may involve as little as a weekend seminar in, for instance, aromatherapy or as much as a four-year medical school program, as in the case of osteopathic medicine.

One question to ask is whether a practitioner graduated from an accredited educational program. Accreditation is similar to certification in that it is a voluntary, nongovernmental process that attests certain standards have been met. Certification, however, evaluates people, while accreditation evaluates institutions, agencies, and educational programs. To determine whether accreditation is meaningful, ask whether the agency granting the accreditation follows the guidelines of the U.S. Department of Education and whether it requires on-site inspection by a team of independent experts, an extensive self-evaluation report, and evaluation by an independent commission.

Keep in mind that sometimes a particular therapy may be so small and specialized that it isn't reasonable to expect its training course to be accredited. For example, Reflexology programs do not have accreditation. In such cases, it's up to you to decide whether you feel confident that a therapist's education and experience is adequate.

PRACTICE REQUIREMENTS

Although the laws are constantly changing, the following is a list of practicing requirements for various disciplines. Remember, not all states have licensure for massage therapy, so when that is mentioned as a requirement, it only applies in states that have licensure.

Some of the following disciplines require one to be licensed as a massage therapist in order to perform it. That is, while a specific specialty may not be licensed, one may need a massage therapy license in order to perform it; for example, there is no license that exists for sports massage, but one needs a massage therapy license to practice sports massage if massage is licensed in that jurisdiction. In this case, a consumer may want to select a licensed massage therapist who also has a certificate in that specialty. But remember, not all certifications are equal. To further complicate things, some states may require one to be licensed in massage therapy in order to perform the therapy, but another state may not.

Alexander Technique

The practice of the Alexander Technique is not licensed. The North American Society of Teachers of the Alexander Technique certifies practitioners who complete 1,600 hours of training, with 80 percent of that training hands-on practice.

Applied Kinesiology

The practice of applied kinesiology is not licensed. The International College of Applied Kinesiology certifies practitioners who complete its 100-hour training program.

Aromatherapy Massage

The practice of aromatherapy by itself is not licensed, nor does it require certification. If used in massage, however, a license is required in states that have massage therapy licensure.

Aston-Patterning

The practice of teaching Aston-Patterning is not licensed. The Aston Training Center certifies practitioners who complete its training program.

Chiropractic Medicine

The practice of chiropractic medicine is licensed in all 50 states and the District of Columbia. Practicing chiropractic without a license anywhere in the United States is illegal.

Craniosacral Therapy

The practice of craniosacral therapy is not licensed, nor does it require certification. The most respected source of education in craniosacral therapy is the Upledger Institute, which offers a progressive series of training courses for practitioners who are licensed or certified in other health-care disciplines, such as chiropractic and massage therapy.

Feldenkrais Method

The practice of the Feldenkrais Method is not licensed. The Feldenkrais Guild certifies practitioners in Feldenkrais, Functional Integration, and Awareness Through Movement. The total program for certification involves 800 or more hours of education.

Hellerwork

The practice of Hellerwork is not licensed. Hellerwork International certifies practitioners who complete its training. (Hellerwork represents another gray area in the law; a massage therapy license may be required in states that have massage therapy licensure.)

Infant Massage

A massage therapy license is required in states that have massage therapy licensure. The International Association of Infant Massage certifies teachers of infant massage who attend its training seminar and pass an examination. Certified teachers instruct parents, caretakers, health-care workers, and others in how to perform infant massage. The practice of infant massage on one's own child is not licensed and does not require certification.

Manual Lymph Drainage

A massage therapy license is required in states that have massage therapy licensure. The practice of manual lymph drainage is not licensed. The Dr. Vodder School certifies practitioners who complete an intensive month-long training course and pass an examination.

Myofascial Release

A massage therapy license is required in states that have massage therapy licensure. The practice of myofascial release is not licensed, nor does it require certification. The source of education in myofascial release is the Myofascial Release (MFR) Treatment Center & Seminars, established by MFR founder John Barnes. The seminars offer a progressive series of training courses, generally aimed at practitioners who already are licensed or certified in other health-care disciplines, such as physical therapy and massage therapy.

On-Site Massage

A massage therapy license is required in states that have massage therapy licensure. The practice may also be further regulated by individual municipalities' health codes and zoning laws. It is not legal in all places, so check with your local government office.

Oriental/Eastern Massage

The practice of various forms of Oriental/Eastern massage is not licensed, nor is certification required. However, various educational organizations, such as the Acupressure Institute, offer certification based on completion of their training program; check with individual programs to determine their requirements for certification. Also, the American Oriental Bodywork Therapy Association certifies practitioners who have completed at least 500 hours of study in Oriental bodywork. (Some practices in this category do require a massage therapy license in states that have massage therapy licensure.)

Osteopathic Medicine

The practice of osteopathic medicine is licensed in all 50 states and the District of Columbia. Practicing osteopathic medicine without a license anywhere in the United States is illegal.

Physical Therapy

The practice of physical therapy is licensed in all 50 states and the District of Columbia. Practicing physical therapy without a license anywhere in the United States is illegal.

Polarity Therapy

The practice of polarity therapy is not licensed. The American Polarity Therapy Association certifies practitioners who have completed 460 hours of training in polarity therapy.

Reflexology

Some states do and some don't require a massage therapy license for performing reflexology. There's some debate about whether reflexology is a form of massage therapy or not. Some massage therapists are also trained in reflexology and they have hundreds of hours of training. Some reflexologists do only reflexology and have only 100 hours training. The practice of reflexology is not licensed, nor is certification required. However, voluntary certification is offered by the American Reflexology Certification Board to those who have completed 100 hours of study and pass an examination.

Reiki

The practice of reiki is not licensed, nor is certification required. However, to become a reiki master, a practitioner must undergo a progressive series of initiations by those who are already masters.

Rolfing

The practice of Rolfing is not licensed. The Rolf Institute certifies practitioners who complete its training program, which involves 650 hours of education. (Rolfing represents a gray area in the law; a massage therapy license may be required in states that have massage therapy licensure.)

Sports Massage

A massage therapy license is required in states that have massage therapy licensure. The American Massage Therapy Association certifies practitioners in sports massage, based on specialized training and written and practical exams.

CRUCIAL QUESTIONS

To help you in choosing a practitioner, here are some questions to ask.

Training and Credentials

* Does the state require licensing in this profession and if so, is the practitioner licensed?
* If licensing is not required, is the practitioner certified? If so, by whom, and is that organization certified? What are the requirements for certification?
* What sort of education and training has the practitioner undergone and for how long? Is the training program accredited and if so, by whom?
* How long has the practitioner been in practice?

Professional Affiliations

* Is the practitioner a member of a recognized nonprofit professional organization? Can the practitioner give you the address of that organization, and is he in fact registered with the group?
* What are the requirements for membership in the organization? Must certain standards be met or are the members required only to pay a fee to join?
* Does the organization have a written code of ethics and standards of practice?
* Does the organization have a system for registering complaints, as well as a disciplinary process?

Financial Matters

* Is the treatment reimbursed by your health insurer? Does referral from a physician enhance the chances of reimbursement?
* What is the cost of a session? How many sessions are likely to be necessary for successful treatment?
* Does the practitioner have malpractice insurance?

Personal Matters

* Do you feel comfortable with the practitioner?
* Was the practitioner willing to answer your questions? Did she outline a clear treatment program?
* What is the practitioner's attitude toward conventional medical treatment you may be receiving? Is that attitude acceptable to you?
* Did the practitioner attempt to diagnose your condition? Unless permitted under licensing laws, this is illegal.

States that License Massage Therapists

Alabama	Louisiana	Oregon
Arkansas	Maine	Rhode Island
Connecticut	Maryland	South Carolina
Delaware	Nebraska	Tennessee
District of	New Hampshire	Texas
Columbia	New Mexico	Utah
Florida	New York	Virginia
Hawaii	North Dakota	Washington
Iowa	Ohio	West Virginia

Therapeutic Touch

The practice of Therapeutic Touch is not licensed, nor is certification required.

Trager Approach

The practice of the Trager Approach is not licensed. The Trager Institute certifies practitioners who complete its training program, which involves 500 hours of education.

Trigger Point Therapy (Neuromuscular and Myotherapy)

A massage therapy license is required of practitioners in states that have massage therapy licensure. The practice of trigger point therapy is not licensed. There are various instructors of neuromuscular therapy and several have their own certification system. Bonnie Prudden Pain Erasure certifies practitioners in Bonnie Prudden Myotherapy after completion of more than 1,000 hours of training. Other forms of trigger point therapy do not necessarily require certification; they may be taught as part of massage school curriculum or in various seminars.

How to Give a Massage

Satisfying our need for touch doesn't necessarily mean paying a visit to a professional. Giving a massage is one of the nicest things family and friends can do for one another. It loosens stiff, sore muscles, reduces stress, enhances immunity, and prompts the body to release endorphins, which are natural opiate-like chemicals that alleviate pain and produce a sense of well-being.

Anyone, young or old, can benefit from giving and receiving massage. And while some people may have an innate talent for the healing art, it can easily be learned. Massage classes and videos are perhaps the best way to learn the different strokes, but you also can give a good massage by following the steps below.

PREPARING THE SPACE

* Choose a quiet time, and eliminate all distractions. Turn off the telephone and the television. If there are other people around, ask them not to disturb you.
* You can give a massage just about anywhere but it's easiest if there is a place for your partner to lie flat and for you to move comfortably all the way around him or her. Be sure the room is warm, and dim the lighting.

Candles are a good way to set a relaxing mood.
* Do not use a bed for massage because it is too soft and doesn't offer the receiver enough support. If you do not have a massage table, have your partner to lie on the floor on a towel placed over a rug or blanket. A futon is also acceptable.
* Provide a bolster or pillow for your partner to place under his knees while lying on his back and under his feet while lying on his stomach. This will help reduce strain on the lower back.

BEFORE YOU BEGIN

* The receiver should remove jewelry, makeup, glasses and contact lenses.
* You should also remove any jewelry. Hands should be clean and nails should be short and smooth. Wear

The Healing Power of Touch

loose-fitting clothes that don't restrict movement. Avoid wearing perfume or cologne, because it might smell unpleasant to your partner and interfere with relaxation.

* Give your partner privacy to disrobe. Leave a sheet and properly sized towel so he can cover himself before you enter the room.

* Select the oil you want to use. Mineral oil, including baby oil, is not easily absorbed and tends to simply sit on the surface of the skin. Instead, use a light vegetable oil, such as almond, grapeseed, or apricot or peach kernel oil. Other choices include avocado, wheatgerm, and jojoba oils. However, these oils are a bit heavier and you may prefer to mix them with almond or grapeseed.

* Vegetable oils can be used plain or mixed with essential oils, which have different effects on the emotions, depending on the oil. Relaxing scents include lavender, chamomile, and neroli. Stimulating oils include lemon, peppermint, and rosemary. Because scent is so personal, ask your partner what aroma he or she prefers. Use two or three drops of essential oil per tablespoon of vegetable oil. (Before using essential oils, however, read the cautions on page 38.)

* Setting a time limit for the massage can be helpful, so that you don't become too tired and your partner isn't wondering when the massage will end. Sixty minutes is fine; 90 minutes is usually the maximum.

THE MASSAGE

* Both you and your partner should take a few deep breaths. Inhale slowly through the nose and exhale through the mouth. This helps you feel calm and centered.

* Keep your partner covered with the sheet, exposing only the area you are working on. Breasts and genitals should not be massaged.

* Rather than pouring oil directly onto your partner's skin, pour a dime-size amount into your hand, then rub it between your palms to warm it.

* Begin the massage with effleurage, which means "touching lightly." This smooth, gliding stroke is done in the direction of the heart. Massage always begins with effleurage, to warm and

CONTRAINDICATIONS

There are a number of instances in which massage should not be performed.

✽ Massage during pregnancy can be very helpful for alleviating a variety of discomforts. However, as with any medical therapy, massage should not be given to a pregnant woman without first clearing it with her doctor. Avoid massaging the abdomen and use only gentle, not deep, pressure on all other areas of the body. Do not use essential oils during pregnancy without the advice of a medical practitioner thoroughly trained in their use.

✽ Do not massage directly on bruises, cuts, sprains, new scar tissue, inflamed or swollen areas, or other injuries. Gentle massage around the area, however, can be beneficial, helping to stimulate circulation and carry away waste products.

✽ Do not perform massage on anyone with heart disease or high blood pressure. Though massage can be beneficial for these conditions, it is best left to a professional.

✽ Do not massage someone who has phlebitis or other circulatory problems, because of the possibility that a blood clot may be released.

✽ Massage of cancer patients is also best left to professionals, given that there is a lot of controversy over whether massage can promote the spread of tumors.

✽ Do not massage any area where a skin condition is present.

relax the muscles and to allow the giver to feel any areas of tension. If at any point you feel unsure of yourself, return to effleurage.

✽ Once the muscles are warmed up, you can proceed to kneading, a movement that is much like kneading bread dough. Alternately squeeze and roll the muscles between your hands. Be sure to use enough oil to avoid pinching the skin. Kneading is best done on fleshy areas, such as the thighs and buttocks, but it also works well on the shoulders, upper arms, and lower legs.

✽ Use pressure that is as firm as your partner likes. Some strokes to try are wringing, or pushing along the muscles with one hand as you pull with the opposite hand; firm, spreading motions with the thumbs or palms; and circling motions with one or both hands spread flat.

❋ Avoid applying pressure to bony areas, and do not exert pressure directly on the spinal column.

❋ A nice way to end a massage is by using the fingertips to gently stroke all parts of the body with feathering motions, alternating one hand after the other.

AFTER A MASSAGE

❋ Leave your partner alone to rest for a few minutes. Tell him to take his time getting up.

❋ To reduce stress on the spine, have your partner roll onto his side before rising, using his arms to push himself up.

❋ Your partner should be sure to drink several glasses of water in the hours following a massage, to help the body eliminate toxins that have been released.

❋ Both of you should set aside time to rest for an hour or so afterward. Giving a massage can be draining, and you need time to refresh yourself, perhaps by drinking some herbal tea or taking a bath. Your partner will probably feel deeply relaxed after the massage; to avoid spoiling its effects, he should avoid rushing off to some busy activity.

Appendix/Resources

Acupressure

Acupressure Institute
1533 Shattuck Ave.
Berkeley, CA 94709
800-442-2232
Conducts acupressure training,
certifies practitioners, and
provides general information.

American Association of
    Oriental Medicine
433 Front St.
Catasauqua, PA 18032
610-266-1433
Professional organization for
practitioners. Provides referrals
to members.

Alexander Technique

American Center for the
    Alexander Technique
129 W. 67th St.
New York, NY 10023
212-799-0468
The oldest training center for
the Alexander Technique in
the United States.

North American Society of
    Teachers of the Alexander
    Technique
3010 Hennepin Ave. South
Suite 10
Minneapolis, MN 55408
800-473-0620
Professional organization for
practitioners. Provides training,

certification, information, and
referrals.

Applied Kinesiology

International College of
    Applied Kinesiology
6405 Metcalf Ave., Suite 503
Shawnee Mission, KS
66202-3929
913-384-5336
Web site: www.icak.com
Provides information and
referrals.

Touch for Health Association
3223 Washington
Marina Del Rey, CA 90292
310-574-7833

Aromatherapy

American Herb Association
P.O. Box 2482
Nevada City, CA 95959
916-265-9552

National Association for
    Holistic Aromatherapy
P.O. Box 17622
Boulder, CO 80308
800-566-6735
Offers aromatherapy classes
and provides referrals.

Aston-Patterning

Aston Training Center
P.O. Box 489
Incline Village, NV 89450
702-831-8228

e-mail: astonpat@aol.com
Trains and certifies practioners.
Provides referrals.

Ayurvedic Medicine

Ayurvedic Institute
11311 Menaul N.E.
Albuquerque, NM 87112
505-291-9698
Web site: www.ayurveda.com
Provides training in Ayurvedic
medicine and other general
information.

The Raj
1734 Jasmine Ave.
Fairfield, IA 52556-9005
515-472-5866
A spa that provides treatments
based on Maharishi Ayur
Veda.

Chiropractic

American Chiropractic
  Association
1701 Clarendon Blvd.
Arlington, VA 22209
703-276-8800
Web site: www.amerchiro.org
Professional organization.
Provides general information
and referrals.

The World Chiropractic
  Alliance
2950 N. Dobson
Suite 1
Chandler, AZ 85224
800-347-1011
Professional organization.

Craniosacral Therapy

Cranial Academy
8606 Allisonville Road,
Suite 130
Indianapolis, IN 46250
317-594-0411
Web site:
www.rhemamed.com/ca.htm
Professional organization for
practitioners of cranial
osteopathy.

Upledger Institute
11211 Prosperity Farms Road,
Suite D-325
Palm Beach Gardens, FL
33410-3487
800-233-5880
Web site: www.upledger.com
An education, resource, and
treatment center.

Feldenkrais Method

Feldenkrais Guild
706 Ellsworth St. S.W.
Albany, OR 97321
800-775-2118
Web site: www.feldenkrais.com
Trains and certifies practitioners and provides referrals.

Hellerwork

Hellerwork International
406 Berry St.
Mt. Shasta, CA 96067
916-926-2500
Offers training and certification
for practitioners and provides
information and referrals for
the general public.

Infant Massage

International Association of
  Infant Massage
1720 Willow Creek Circle,
Suite 516
Eugene, OR 97402
800-248-5432
Provides information and
trains and certifies instructors
of infant massage.

Jin Shin Do

Jin Shin Do Foundation for
  Bodymind Acupressure
1084G San Miguel Canyon
Road
Watsonville, CA 95076
408-763-7702
Trains practitioners and pro-
vides information.

Jin Shin Jyutsu

Jin Shin Jyutsu, Inc.
8719 E. San Alberto
Scottsdale, AZ 85258
602-998-9331
Trains practitioners and provides information.

Manual Lymph Drainage

North American Vodder
  Association of Lymphatic
  Therapy (NAVALT)
P.O. Box 861
Chesterland, OH 44026
888-462-8258
Provides information and
referrals.

Dr. Vodder School
  North America
P.O. Box 5701
Victoria, British Columbia
Canada
250-598-9862
Training school for
practitioners.

Massage Therapy

American Massage Therapy
  Association
820 Davis St., Suite 100
Evanston, IL 60201-4444
847-864-0123
Web site:
www.amtamassage.org
Professional organization for
certified practitioners. Provides
general information.

Associated Bodywork &
  Massage Professionals
28677 Buffalo Park Road
Evergreen, CO 80439
800-458-2267 or
303-674-0859
Web site: www.abmp.com
Professional organization.
Provides general information.

Myofascial Release

Myofascial Release Treatment
  Centers and Seminars
10 S. Leopard Road, Suite 1
Paoli, PA 19301-1569
800-FASCIAL
Web site:
vll.com/MFR/index.html
Provides seminar information.

Myotherapy

Bonnie Prudden Pain Erasure
7800 W. Speedway
Tucson, AZ 85710
800-221-4634
Offers treatment programs.
Certifies practitioners and
provides referrals.

Osteopathic Medicine

American Academy of
    Osteopathy
3500 DePauw Blvd.
Suite 1081
Indianapolis, IN 46268-1136
317-879-1881
Web site:
www.rhemamed.com/aao.htm
Professional organization.

American Osteopathic
    Association
142 E. Ontario St.
Chicago, IL 60611
800-621-1773
Web site:
www.am-osteo-assn.org/
index.htm
Professional organization.

Physical Therapy

American Physical Therapy
    Association
1111 N. Fairfax St.
Alexandria, VA 22314
703-684-APTA
Web site: www.apta.org
Professional organization.
Publishes the scientific journal
Physical Therapy.

Polarity Therapy

American Polarity Therapy
    Association
2888 Bluff St., Suite 149
Boulder, CO 80301
303-545-2080
Professional organization that
certifies practitioners.

Polarity Wellness Center
10 Leonard St., Suite A
New York, NY 10013
212-334-8392
Provides information, publications, and referrals for the
general public.

Reflexology

International Institute of
    Reflexology
P.O. Box 12642
St. Petersburg, FL
33733-2642
813-343-4811

Reiki

The Reiki Alliance
P.O. Box 41
Cataldo, ID 83810
208-682-3535

Rolfing

Rolf Institute
205 Canyon Blvd.
Boulder, CO 80306-1868
303-449-5903 or
800-530-8875
e-mail: RolfInst@aol.com
Training center that certifies
practitioners. Offers books and

informational literature, as well as a list of certified practitioners across the country.

Shiatsu

American Oriental Bodywork Therapy Association
Laurel Oak Corporate Center, Suite 408
1010 Haddonfield-Berlin Road
Voorhees, NJ 08043
609-782-1616
Professional organization that certifies practitioners.

Sports Massage

American Massage Therapy Association
820 Davis St., Suite 100
Evanston, IL 60201-4444
847-864-0123
Web site:
www.amtamassage.org
Offers practitioner certification in sports massage.

Therapeutic Touch

Nurse Healers—Professional Associates, Inc.
1211 Locust St.
Philadelphia, PA 19107
215-545-8079
Organization for health professionals.

Orcas Island Foundation
Box 86, Route 1
East Sound, WA 98245
360-376-4526
Offers workshops on Therapeutic Touch.

Pumpkin Hollow Farm
Box 135, RR 1
Craryville, NY 12521
518-325-3583
Offers workshops on Therapeutic Touch.

Trager Approach

The Trager Institute
21 Locust Ave.
Mill Valley, CA 94941
415-388-2688
Provides training and certification for practitioners and offers information and referrals for the general public.

Tui-Na

American Oriental Bodywork Therapy Association
Laurel Oak Corporate Center, Suite 408
1010 Haddonfield-Berlin Road
Voorhees, NJ 08043
609-782-1616
Professional organization that certifies practitioners.

INDEX

A

accreditation, 234

acne, 39

acupressure, 28–30. *See also* Jin Shin Do; tui-na.
    arthritis, 128
    asthma, 131
    bladder infections, 139
    cancer, 150
    carpal tunnel syndrome, 152
    chemotherapy, 24, 30
    chronic fatigue syndrome, 154
    chronic pain, 157
    colic, 159
    colitis, 161
    dental pain, 30
    foot pain, 179
    headaches, 181
    hypertension, 185
    insomnia, 187
    leg cramps, 195
    menstrual pain, 194
    nausea and vomiting, 24, 30, 202
    postsurgical recovery, 202
    pregnancy, 24, 30, 185, 204, 225
    sciatica, 209
    sinusitis, 213
    temporomandibular disorder (TMD), 225
    tinnitus, 229

AIDS (acquired immunodeficiency syndrome). *See* HIV/AIDS.

Alexander Technique, 31–32
    carpal tunnel syndrome, 153
    tendinitis, 228
    uses, 32–33

allergies, 130

anxiety, 124–125. *See also* stress.

aromatherapy massage, 39–40
    conventional treatment, 125
    Rolfing, 24
    touch therapy, 126

applied kinesiology, 6, 34–35
    burns, 147
    sports injuries, 215
    sprains and strains, 218
    tendinitis, 215, 227
    uses, 36

aromatherapy massage, 37–39
    anxiety, 126, 175, 204
    asthma, 131
    back pain, 135
    bladder infections, 139
    burns, 145
    bursitis, 148
    cancer, 150
    chronic fatigue syndrome, 154–155
    chronic pain, 157
    colitis, 161
    constipation, 166
    depression, 168, 175
    fibromyalgia, 175–176
    headaches, 181
    HIV/AIDS, 123
    hypertension, 185
    indigestion, 203
    insomnia, 175–176, 187
    menopause, 192
    menstrual pain, 194
    muscle cramps and tension, 195
    muscle pain, 175, 215, 218
    nausea and vomiting, 197, 203
    postsurgical recovery, 203
    pregnancy, 204–205
    premenstrual syndrome (PMS), 202
    pre-surgery, 204
    sinusitis, 213
    sports injuries, 215
    sprains and strains, 218
    stress, 221
    tendinitis, 227
    uses, 39–40